Local Treatment of Inflammatory Joint Diseases

Willm Uwe Kampen • Manfred Fischer

Editors

Local Treatment of Inflammatory Joint Diseases

Benefits and Risks

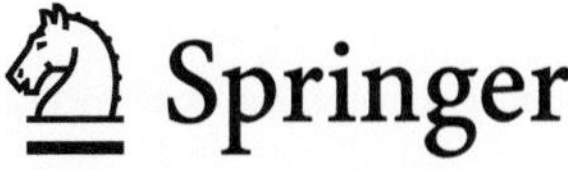 Springer

Editors
Willm Uwe Kampen
Nuklearmedizin Spitalerhof
Hamburg, Germany

Manfred Fischer
Kassel, Germany

ISBN 978-3-319-35022-6 ISBN 978-3-319-16949-1 (eBook)
DOI 10.1007/978-3-319-16949-1

Printed on acid-free paper

Springer International Publishing AG Switzerland is part of Springer Science+Business Media
(www.springer.com)

Preface

More than 60 years ago, in 1952, Fellinger and Schmid published data about intra-articular administration of either 3.7–7.4 MBq ^{131}I or 37 MBq ^{198}Au. They observed a significant reduction of pain in patients suffering from rheumatoid arthritis (1).

Today three radionuclides are approved and/or sold in many countries (Table 1) for treatment of inflammatory joint diseases. The aim of radiosynovectomy is to decrease swelling, pain, stiffness and joint effusion to improve joint function by treating inflammation of synovial tissue using β-emitting radiocolloids.

Although many studies have proven its therapeutic efficacy and safety and many thousands of successful treatments are done by experienced nuclear medicine physicians, assuming both a responsible and proper patient selection and a skilful injection technique, there is still a controversial discussion about its benefits and risks.

In patients suffering from inflammatory joint diseases, synovium shows thickening of the lining layer, increased vascularity and inflammatory cell infiltration

Table 1 Approval and Disposal of radionclides used for radiosynovectomy

	^{90}Yttrium	^{186}Rhenium	^{169}Erbium
Country	Approval	Approval	Approval
Germany	x	x	x
France	x	x	x
Switzerland	x	x	x
Portugal	x		
Belgium	x		
Netherlands	x		
Luxembourg	x		
Greece	x		
Norway	x		
Irland	x		
Turkey	x	x	x
Czech Rep.	x	x	x
Mexico	x	x	x
Approval vs. sales	Approved in 13 countries Sold in 28 countries	Approved in 6 countries Sold in 16 countries	Approved in 6 countries Sold in 14 countries

in a wide heterogeneity. Multiple factors, mechanical and biochemical, are responsible for structural changes of synovial membrane, cartilage, subchondral bone, ligaments and periarticular muscles. Higher levels of osteogenic protein1, hyaluronic acid, cytokines and others may be detected in synovial fluid in inflammatory joint diseases. The relationship between these factors and inflammatory mediators and their contribution to changes in different joint tissues in inflammatory joint diseases may influence therapeutic results. To delay or even to avoid progression of structural changes needs multi-/interdisciplinary therapy including radiosynovectomy.

The indication for RSO is given, if the expected benefit for the patient overweights the possible risks and if no other treatment option does have an advantageous risk-benefit ratio.

The major concern of this book is to compare radiation synovectomy to other therapeutic options in case of local synovitis, like systemic pharmacological therapy, intra-articular corticosteroid injections or surgery. Independently from the modality used, each treatment may be hampered by adverse reactions or adverse events. Knowing benefit and risk of different therapeutic modalities is mandatory for safety of patients.

The editors are happy that internationally well-known colleagues agreed to contribute to this book and we like to thank them for their valuable input. We learned a lot working for this book and we would be happy if the readers would agree with us.

Hamburg, Germany   Willm Uwe Kampen
Kassel, Germany   Manfred Fischer

Contents

Safety of Medicines: Detection and Reporting Adverse Reactions

Manfred Fischer, Annette Brinker, and Barbara Sickmüller

Contents

This chapter describes the definitions of adverse reactions/events, pharmacovigilance systems, their limitations and basic problems, as well as adverse events connected with radiopharmaceutical agents.

M. Fischer (✉)
Institute of Radiology, Radiation Therapy and Nuclear Medicine, Friedrich-Ebert-Str.
D-34117, 55 Kassel, Germany
e-mail: finukskk@aol.com

A. Brinker
Brinker Pharmaconsulting, Stölpchen Weg D-14109, 37 Berlin, Germany
e-mail: annettebrinker@brinkerpharma.de

B. Sickmüller
Bundesverband Pharmazeutischer Industrie, Willemerstrasse D-63067, 11 Offenbach, Germany
e-mail: b.sickmueller@advisor.bpi.de

© Springer International Publishing Switzerland 2015
W.U. Kampen, M. Fischer (eds.), *Local Treatment of Inflammatory Joint Diseases: Benefits and Risks*, DOI 10.1007/978-3-319-16949-1_1

1.1   Introduction

For developing a new medicinal product[1], preclinical studies and phase I, phase II and phase III clinical trials have to be performed for obtaining marketing authorisations[2] from regulatory authorities. In preclinical studies as well as in phase I, II and III clinical trials, it is impossible to identify all safety concerns. This is because of the study design, which is primarily aimed at the proof of efficacy of the new substance in selected patient groups. Hence, a study design per se can limit the knowledge about a new therapeutic approach and even more so the risk-benefit balance. In the post-authorisation phase, increasing numbers of patients with co-morbid conditions and treated with concomitant medicinal products are exposed with the new product. Before prescribing a medicinal product, the balance between the product's benefit and risks has to be defined. Therefore, a system of spontaneous reporting of suspected adverse reactions, post-authorisation studies and/or other observational data are important to evaluate the product's risk and to minimise it.

The establishment of the International Drug Monitoring Program from the World Health Organization (WHO) was triggered as a response to the thalidomide adverse reactions, detected in 1961. At that time, thousands of congenital deformed children were born as the result of the intrauterine exposure of an unsafe drug, prescribed to pregnant women. Any drug may cause an adverse drug reaction. According to the US General Accounting Office, in 1990, 51 % of approved medicinal products had serious adverse effects undetected before their approval.

An international system for monitoring adverse drug reactions (ADRs) using information derived from member states was established by the World Health Organization (WHO) in 1971. 'For an effective international system to become effective, an international common reporting form was developed, guidelines for entering information adopted, common technologies and classifications prepared'.

The WHO thought that pharmacovigilance was necessary, because the information about benefit and risk of a new substance collected during the pre-authorisation phase by animal and also human studies was insufficiently predictive to determine human safety. For multinationally approved medicinal products, pharmacovigilance is necessary in each country due to differences in production including pharmaceutical quality, composition, distribution and use of the medicinal product, as well as the specific genetics, diet and tradition of the populations concerned. The WHO system was started with ten countries that had already established national systems for spontaneous ADR reporting.

At the end of 2010, 134 countries were part of this WHO PV Program [1] (Fig. 1.1).

Pharmacovigilance (PV) is defined by WHO as the science and activities relating to the detection, assessment, understanding and prevention of adverse effects or any other medicinal product-related problem. WHO declared the following aims of pharmacovigilance:

---

[1] In European law instead of 'drug', the term 'medicinal product' is used.

[2] In the USA, the term 'drug approval' is used; in Europe the term 'marketing authorisation'.

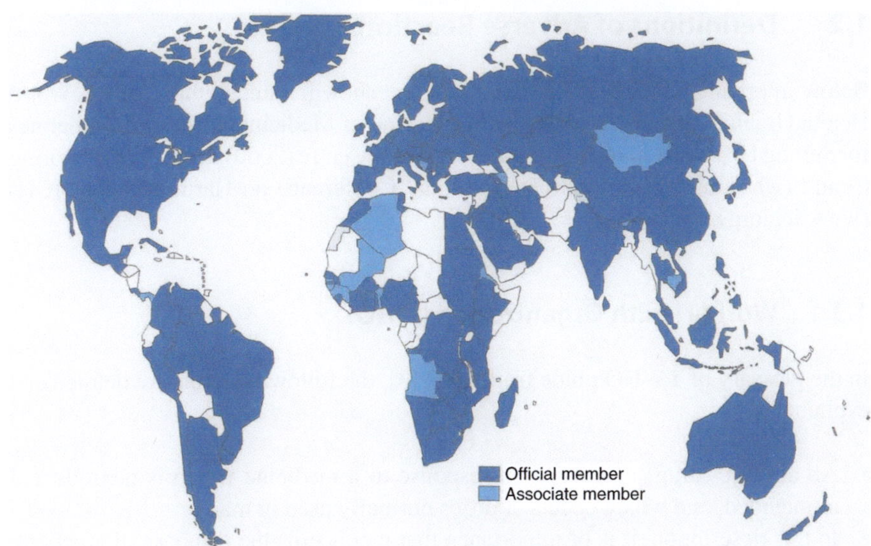

Fig. 1.1 Countries in the WHO Programme for International Drug Monitoring in December 2010 [2]

- 'Early detection of hitherto unknown adverse reactions and interactions
- Detection of increases in frequency of (known) adverse reactions
- Identification of risk factors and possible mechanisms underlying adverse reactions
- Estimation of quantitative aspects of benefit/risk analysis and dissemination needed to improve drug prescribing and regulation.'

The aims of pharmacovigilance are to enhance patient care and patient safety in relation to the use of medicines and to support public health programmes, by providing reliable information for effective assessment of the benefit-risk profile of medicinal products.

The WHO has a mandate from its Member States to develop, establish and promote international standards with respect to food, biological, pharmaceutical and similar products and the provision to adopt regulations concerning standards, with respect to safety, purity and potency of them in international commerce [1].

All medicinal products are subject to an assessment of their quality, efficacy and safety before receiving marketing authorisations. After having been placed on the market, these products continue to be monitored by the marketing authorisation holder and agencies, to assure that any aspect which could impact the safety profile of a medicine is detected and assessed and necessary measures are taken.

Post-authorisation safety monitoring is an important tool for the protection of public health, in respect to novel medicinal products as well as for those having been in the market already for a long time.

1.2   Definitions of Adverse Reactions/Events

Below internationally accepted definitions are shown, namely, those of the World Health Organization (WHO): Safety Monitoring of Medicinal Products: Guidelines for Setting Up and Running a Pharmacovigilance Centre (2000), Uppsala Monitoring Centre (who-umc.org) and the International Conference on Harmonisation (ICH) (www.ich.org).

1.2.1   World Health Organization (WHO)

In the glossary of a WHO guide from 2002 [3], the following terms are defined and explained:

- An adverse (drug) reaction is 'a response to a medicine which is noxious and unintended, and which occurs at doses normally used in man'.
- In this description, it is of importance that it concerns the response of a patient, in which individual factors may play an important role, and that the phenomenon is noxious (an unexpected therapeutic response, e.g. may be a side effect but not an adverse reaction). An unexpected adverse reaction is 'an adverse reaction, the nature or severity of which is not consistent with domestic labeling or market authorisation, or expected from characteristics of the drug'.
- A drug or medicine is 'a pharmaceutical product, used in or on the human body for the prevention, diagnosis or treatment of a disease, or for the modification of physiological functions'.
- A side effect is 'any unintended effect of a pharmaceutical product occurring at doses normally used by a patient which is related to the pharmacological proper-ties of the drug'. Essential elements in this definition are the pharmaceutical nature of the effect that the phenomenon is unintended and that there is no delib-erated overdose.
- An adverse event or experience is defined as 'any untoward medical occurrence that may present during treatment with a medicine but which does not necessar-ily have a causal relationship with the treatment'. The basic point here is the coincidence in time without any suspicion of a causal relationship with this treatment.

The Uppsala Monitoring Centre differentiates adverse reactions in different groups:

- Type A effects are 'drug actions', due to overreaction on pharmacological effects and dose related; interactions between medicinal products, especially pharmaco-kinetic interactions, may often be classified as Type A effects.
- Type B 'patients' reactions' occurring in patients with predisposed conditions (immunological or non-immunological effects); they are generally rare and unpredictable.

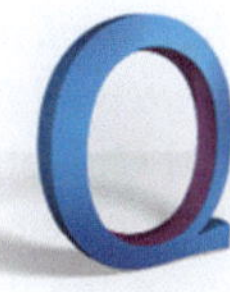
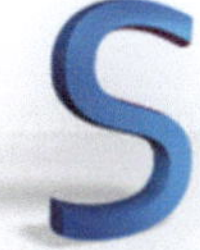
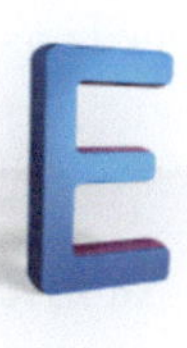

Fig. 1.2 ICH Guideline. The topics are divided into four categories and ICH topic codes are designed according to these categories

- Type C effects 'refer to situations in which the frequency of "spontaneous" diseases is enhanced'. This 'may have pronounced effects on public health'.

With these 'ABC groups', practically all medicine-related problems can be classified, taking into account their characteristics and distinctions. This system distinguishes between appropriate and inappropriate drug use, dose-related and dose-unrelated problems and types A ('drug actions'), B ('patient reactions') and C ('statistical') adverse effects. This classification may serve as an educational tool and may be useful when choosing a study method and for the design of effective strategies in pharmacovigilance [4].

1.2.2   International Conference on Harmonisation: ICH

The International Conference on Harmonisation of Technical Requirements for Registration of Pharmaceuticals for Human Use (ICH) started in 1990 and brings together the regulatory authorities and pharmaceutical industry of Europe, Japan and the USA to discuss scientific and technical aspects of drug registration. From the beginning, WHO, the European EFTA States, represented by Switzerland, and Canada had observer status. ICH's first decade saw significant progress in the development of Tripartite ICH Guidelines on Safety (S), Quality (Q) and Efficacy (E) topics (Fig. 1.2).

Work was also undertaken on a number of important multidisciplinary topics (M), which included MedDRA (Medical Dictionary for Regulatory Activities – M1) and Electronic Transmission of Individual Case Safety Reports Message Specification (M2 ICSR (R2)).

- *Post-Approval Safety Data Management: Definitions and Standards for Expedited Reporting (Current Version Dated 12 November 2003* [5])
  This tripartite harmonised ICH Guideline provides a standardised procedure for post-approval safety data management including expedited reporting to the relevant authority. The practices of the data management were standardised. Now cases, obtained from consumers, literatures and Internets, were all specific to post-approval data management. Good case management practice was focused and recommended for expedited reporting with clear definitions.
- *Adverse Event (AE)*
  An adverse event is any untoward medical occurrence in a patient administered a medicinal product and which does not necessarily have to have a causal relationship with this treatment. An adverse event can therefore be any unfavourable and unintended sign (e.g. an abnormal laboratory finding), symptom or disease temporally associated with the use of a medicinal product, whether or not considered related to this medicinal product.
- *Adverse Drug Reaction (ADR)*
  Adverse drug reactions, as established by regional regulations, guidance and practices, concern noxious and unintended responses to a medicinal product.
  The phrase 'responses to a medicinal product' means that a causal relationship between a medicinal product and an adverse event is at least a reasonable possibility [6].
  A reaction, in contrast to an event, is characterised by the fact that a causal relationship between the drug and the occurrence is suspected. For regulatory reporting purposes, if an event is spontaneously reported, even if the relationship is unknown or unstated, it meets the definition of an adverse drug reaction.
- *Serious AE/ADR*
  In accordance with the ICH E2A guideline [6], a serious adverse event or reaction is any untoward medical occurrence that at any dose:
  - Results in death.
  - Is life-threatening (NOTE: the term 'life-threatening' in the definition of 'serious' refers to an event/reaction in which the patient was at risk of death at the time of the event/reaction; it does not refer to an event/ reaction which hypothetically might have caused death if it were more severe).
  - Requires inpatient hospitalisation or results in prolongation of existing hospitalisation.
  - Results in persistent or significant disability/incapacity.
  - Is a congenital anomaly/birth defect.
  - Is a medically important event or reaction. Medical and scientific judgement should be exercised in deciding whether other situations should be considered serious such as important medical events that might not be immediately life-threatening or result in death or hospitalisation but might jeopardise the patient or might require intervention to prevent one of the other outcomes listed in the definition above. Examples of such events are intensive treatment in an emergency room or at home for allergic bronchospasm, blood dyscrasias or convulsions that do not result in hospitalisation or development of drug dependency or drug abuse.

- *Unexpected ADR*
  An ADR whose nature, severity, specificity or outcome is not consistent with the term or description used in the local or regional product labelling (e.g. package insert or summary of product characteristics (SmPC)) should be considered unexpected. When a marketing authorisation holder (MAH) is uncertain whether an ADR is expected or unexpected, the ADR should be treated as unexpected.

  An expected ADR with a fatal outcome should be considered unexpected unless the local/regional product labelling specifically states that the ADR might be associated with a fatal outcome.

1.3   Pharmacovigilance Systems in the European Union (EU) and the USA

1.3.1   EU: Legislation, GCP-Modules and the European Medicines Agency (EMA)

The European Union pharmacovigilance system was revised in 2010 so as to become more effective [7]. The implementation of the new system started in July 2012. It acts at three different hierarchical levels:

- With regard to pharmacovigilance, the European Medicine Agency (EMA) has the main tasks of the management of the Union pharmacovigilance database and data-processing network (the EudraVigilance database), the coordination of safety information coming from Member States and the coordination of information regarding safety issues to the public.
  Within EMA the responsibility lies with the *Pharmacovigilance Risk Assessment Committee (PRAC)*. PRAC is responsible for assessing all aspects of the risk management of medicines for human use. This includes the detection, assessment, minimisation and communication relating to the risk of adverse reactions, while taking the therapeutic effect of the medicine into account. It also has responsibility for the design and evaluation of post-authorisation safety studies and pharmacovigilance audit. Members of the PRAC are nominated by the European Union Member States, in consultation with the Agency's Management Board. They are chosen on the strength of their qualifications and expertise with regard to pharmacovigilance matters and risk assessments of medicines for human use. To represent healthcare professionals and patient organisations, the European Commission appoints two members and two alternates following consultation with the EU Parliament. The European Commission also appoints six independent scientific experts.
- At the second level, each Member State shall designate a competent authority for the performance of its pharmacovigilance responsibilities and shall establish a pharmacovigilance system, to ensure the monitoring and supervision of the medicinal products authorised in their territory and to take appropriate measures

as necessary. They shall perform a regular audit of their pharmacovigilance system and report the results to the EU Commission.

- Finally, the marketing authorisation holders (MAHs) shall establish their own pharmacovigilance system equivalent to the relevant Member State's pharmacovigilance system, to ensure the monitoring and supervision of their authorised medicinal products and to take appropriate measures as necessary. They shall perform a regular audit of their pharmacovigilance system.

Parties being directly involved in pharmacovigilance are:

- Consumers (persons who are not healthcare professionals, such as patients, lawyers, friends, relatives of a patient or carers) are asked to communicate any suspected adverse reaction to his/her doctor, pharmacist, or healthcare professional or directly to the national competent authorities (new standard text in all package leaflets).
- Healthcare professionals (such as physicians, dentists, pharmacists, nurses, medical technologists, all persons working in a medical institution, coroners or as otherwise by local authorities specified persons) are asked to report suspected adverse reactions directly to the national competent authorities (new standard text in all summary of product characteristics (SmPC)).

Consumers and healthcare professionals are free to report to marketing authorisation holders (MAHs) and other distributors of medicinal products.

Based on the new EU Legislation, the European Medicines Agency (EMA) published new definitions in the guidelines on good pharmacovigilance practices [8]. They are very similar to the WHO definitions:

- Adverse reaction (synonyms, adverse drug reaction (ADR), suspected adverse (drug) reaction, adverse effect, undesirable effect): A response to a medicinal product which is noxious and unintended. A response in this context means that a causal relationship between a medicinal product and an adverse event is at least a reasonable possibility. Adverse reactions may arise from use of the product within or outside the terms of the marketing authorisation or from occupational exposure. Conditions of use outside the marketing authorisation include off-label use, overdose, misuse, abuse and medication error.
- Unexpected adverse reaction: An adverse reaction, the nature, severity or outcome of which is not consistent with the summary of product characteristics. This includes class-related reactions which are mentioned in the summary of product characteristics (SmPC) but which are not specifically described as occurring with this product. For products authorised nationally, the relevant SmPC is that authorised by the competent authority in the Member State to whom the reaction is being reported. For centrally authorised products, the relevant SmPC is the SmPC authorised by the European Commission. During the time period

between a Committee for Medicinal Products for Human Use (CHMP) opinion in favour for granting a marketing authorisation and the Commission decision granting the marketing authorisation, the relevant SmPC is the SmPC annexed to the CHMP opinion.

- Adverse event (AE) (synonym, adverse experience): Any untoward medical occurrence in a patient or clinical trial subject administered a medicinal product and which does not necessarily have a causal relationship with this treatment. An adverse event can therefore be any unfavourable and unintended sign (e.g. an abnormal laboratory finding), symptom or disease temporally associated with the use of a medicinal product, whether or not considered related to the medicinal product.
- Serious adverse reaction: An adverse reaction which results in death, is life-threatening, requires inpatient hospitalisation or prolongation of existing hospitalisation, results in persistent or significant disability or incapacity or is a congenital anomaly/birth defect. Medical and scientific judgement should be exercised in deciding whether other situations should be considered serious reactions, such as important medical events that might not be immediately life-threatening or result in death or hospitalisation, but might jeopardise the patient or might require intervention to prevent one of the other outcomes listed above. Any suspected transmission via a medicinal product of an infectious agent is also considered a serious reaction.
- Solicited sources of individual case safety reports: organised data collection systems, which include clinical trials, registries, post-management programmes, surveys of patients or healthcare providers or information gathering on efficacy or patient compliance.
  For the purpose of safety reporting, solicited reports should not be considered spontaneous but classified as Individual Case Safety Reports from studies and therefore should have an appropriate causality assessment by a healthcare professional or the marketing authorisation holder [5].

Information in special situations *with no associated adverse reaction*: the marketing authorisation holder (MAH) has to collect the information and discuss it in the periodic safety update report (PSUR), as applicable):

- Exposure to a medicinal product during pregnancy
- Exposure to a medicinal product during breastfeeding
- Data on use in children
- Reports on compassionate use/named patient use
- Lack of therapeutic efficacy or effect (reports may be required for medicinal products used in critical conditions or for the treatment of life-threatening diseases) reports of medication error
- Administration of products via an incorrect route
- Drug exposure via mother, father or other [9]

1.3.1.1 Special Responsibilities of the Marketing Authorisation Holders (MAHs) and the EU: National Competent Authorities (NCAs)

As part of the pharmacovigilance system, the marketing authorisation holder shall have permanently and continuously an appropriately EU qualified person responsible for pharmacovigilance at his disposal (EU QPPV). If there are additional national contact persons for pharmacovigilance nominated in different EU Member States, their responsibility within the internal pharmacovigilance system and training of the staff has to be defined in the pharmacovigilance system master file (PSMF) [7]. This is controlled by internal audit and inspections by authorities.

If a patient reports a suspected adverse reaction to the marketing authorisation holder, the qualified person for pharmacovigilance shall contact the healthcare professional to get a medical confirmation of the adverse reaction if the patient agrees. All serious adverse reactions have to be reported by the marketing authorisation holder to the health authorities not later than 15 days after the first receipt of the initial report (worldwide). After the full functioning of the EudraVigilance database, in addition all non-serious adverse reactions occurring in the EU will have to be notified to the authorities as individual cases (within 30 days).

It is the responsibility of the national competent authorities and the marketing authorisation holders to have a quality management system in place to ensure compliance with the necessary quality standards at every stage of the documentation of an adverse reaction, such as data collection, data transfer, data management, data coding, case validation, case evaluation, case follow-up, reporting of individual cases (individual case safety report – ICSR) and case archiving.

With the implementation of the new legislation in July 2012, the pharmacovigilance system has to be described in a pharmacovigilance system master file (PSMF), stored at the marketing authorisation holder, ready for inspection at any time by the national competent authorities or the European Medicines Agency (EMA).

Main tasks of the marketing authorisation holders are:

- Collecting, managing and assessment of data on the safety of their medicinal products from reports of patients, healthcare professionals, literature searches and searches in databases of the regulatory agencies.
- Reporting of those data to national competent authorities (NCAs) or the European Medicines Agency (EMA), as applicable periodic safety update reports (PSURs) have to be worked out and reported to EMA [10, 11].
- Signal detection and signal management: the report of the Council for International Organisations of Medical Sciences Working Group VIII Practical Aspects of Signal Detection in Pharmacovigilance [12] defines a signal as *information that arises from one or multiple sources (including observations and experiments), which suggests a new potentially causal association, or a new aspect of a known association, between an intervention and an event or set of related events.* As a general principle, signal detection should follow a recognised methodology, which may vary depending on the type of medicinal product it is intended to cover. Vaccines may, for example, require other methodological strategies [13].

- Implementing Risk Management Plans
- Internal audits to guarantee quality of the PV system
- Information of involved parties and the public
- Regulatory action*s such* as variations, if needed

Risk Management Plan It shall contain a characterisation of the safety profile and an identification of the risks of the medicinal product and depicts all measures and interventions to prevent or minimise those risks and ascertains the effectiveness of the mentioned measures and interventions. Parts of the Risk Management Plan are the safety specification which should be a summary of the identified risks, important potential risks and important missing information and the pharmacovigilance plan, which proposes actions to address the identified safety concerns and includes also the post-authorisation safety studies.

Screening of Literature For the monitoring of the safety profile, literature is an important source. Therefore, reports of suspected adverse reactions from literature should be reviewed and assessed by marketing authorisation holders to identify and record Individual case safety reports, originating either from spontaneous reports or from non-interventional post-authorisation studies.

For the safe use of medicinal products, it is important that physicians publish adverse reactions/experience with a medicinal product in the scientific literature. However, adverse reactions are often published several months after their occurrence. In the context of patient safety, this is rather questionable, as new and important information on ADRs is not available quickly enough to be considered in pharmacovigilance systems. Thus, in order to improve and accelerate the information flow, it is proposed to demand from the authors of case reports that they also report in parallel the adverse reaction/experience to the authorities. This would improve the safety of patients. It would be comparable to the publication of controlled clinical trials. In this case the author would have to provide the registration number in clinical trial registries as part of the checklist for a publication (Consolidated Standards of Reporting Trials (CONSORT) Statement) [14].

Reporting by Member States Competent authorities in Member States shall ensure that all serious Individual Case Safety Reports (ICSRs) that occur in their territory and that are reported to them, including those received from marketing authorisation holders, are made available to the EudraVigilance database.

EudraVigilance adheres to the international safety reporting guidance issued by the International Conference on Harmonisation (ICH) [15]. Adverse reactions and medication errors are coded to terms in the Medical Dictionary for Regulatory Activities (MedDRA) terminology.

In order to facilitate reporting and make it more transparent, it is planned that all reports shall go directly to the European EudraVigilance database as soon as the EMA can assure functioning of the database.

Reporting by EMA The European Medicines Agency shall make available to the WHO Collaborating Centre for International Drug Monitoring all suspected adverse reaction reports occurring in the EU [REG Art 28c(1)] on a weekly basis. It will replace the requirements of Member States participating in the WHO Programme for International Drug Monitoring to directly report to WHO suspected adverse reaction reports occurring in their territory.

The Agency and the European Monitoring Centre for Drugs and Drug Addiction shall also exchange information that they receive on the abuse of medicinal products including information related to illicit drugs [9].

1.3.2 US Laws and Regulations and the Food and Drug Administration (FDA)

The Center for Drug Evaluation and Research (CDER) and the Center for Biologics Evaluation and Research (CBER) of the US Food and Drug Administration (FDA) monitor and review safety information throughout a medicinal product's life cycle, from application for marketing authorisation through approval of the application and after the drug is marketed. The pharmacovigilance system in the USA encompasses all scientific and data-gathering activities relating to the detection, assessment and evaluation of safety signals and includes:

- Safety signal identification
- Pharmacoepidemiologic assessment and safety signal interpretation
- Pharmacovigilance plan development (guidance for industry – good pharmacovigilance practice and pharmacoepidemiologic assessment – March 2005) [16].

1.3.2.1 FDA Adverse Event Reporting System (FAERS)

The FDA Adverse Event Reporting System (FAERS) is a database that contains information on adverse event and medication error reports submitted to the FDA. The database is designed to support the FDA's post-marketing safety surveillance programme for drug and therapeutic biologic products. The informatic structure of the FAERS database adheres to the international safety reporting guidance issued by the International Conference on Harmonisation [15]. Adverse events and medication errors are coded to terms in the Medical Dictionary for Regulatory Activities (MedDRA) terminology.

In the USA reporting of adverse events is voluntarily for healthcare professionals and consumers, including patients themselves, family members and also their lawyers. If these two groups report an adverse event to a drug manufacturer, this one is required to report to the FDA.

In 2013, the 'post-marketing reporting of adverse drug experience' was revised [17], following in most parts the ICH harmonised tripartite guideline, mentioned above, defining in detail:

- Adverse drug experience: adverse event, which is associated with the use of a drug, whether or not considered drug related, including the following: an adverse event occurring in the course of the use of a drug product in professional practice, an adverse event occurring from drug overdose whether accidental or intentional and an adverse event occurring from drug abuse, drug withdrawal and any failure of expected pharmacological action.

- Disability: a substantial disruption of a person's ability to conduct normal life functions
- Life-threatening adverse drug experience: immediate risk of death after administration of a drug.
- Serious adverse drug experience: any adverse drug experience resulting in death, life-threatening reaction, inpatient hospitalisation, prolongation of hospitalisation, disability/incapacity and congenital abnormality/birth defect, independently from the drug's dose administered to the patient. Also serious events are those experiences which may jeopardise a patient and may require any procedure (medication of surgery) to prevent one of the outcomes listed in this definition. Unexpected adverse drug experience: any adverse event which occurs after drug administration, which is not listed in the current labelling of the drug product. This includes events that may be symptomatically and pathophysiologically related to an event listed in the labelling but differ from the event because of greater severity or specificity post-marketing 15-day 'Alert reports': any adverse drug experience, which is both serious and unexpected, whether foreign or domestic, has to be reported as soon as possible after receipt of the information, in no case later than 15 calendar days after receipt. Same deadline is true for any follow-up report. The reporting may be done in paper form or electronically by the drug manufacturer, packer or distributor.
- Scientific literature: a 15-day Alert report based on information from the scientific literature is required to be accompanied by a copy of the published article. The 15-day reporting requirements apply only to reports found in scientific and medical journals either as case reports or as the result of a formal clinical trial.

Evaluation and Mitigation Strategies (REMS): The FDA has the authority to require manufacturers to implement special risk management programmes 'REMS' for their products if the FDA believes such a programme is necessary to assure that the drug's benefits outweigh its risks. REMS programmes utilise tools that go beyond routine labelling. Their requirements may range from the relatively simple, such as education for patients in the form of written information called Medication Guides, to the more complex, such as required training or certification for healthcare providers, patient monitoring, restricting use to particular healthcare settings, requiring medical tests as a condition for dispensing or enrolment in a patient registry [18].

1.3.3   Summary: Pharmacovigilance Systems

In both the EU and the USA, pharmacovigilance activities cover the whole life cycle of medicinal products for human use. The full safety profile of medicinal products can only be known in the marketing period. Therefore, pharmacovigilance activities are especially important for the protection of the patients and public health. As shown above, the definitions and procedures are different in details, but the pharmacovigilance systems in both areas demand expedited and obligational recording and reporting of all available (worldwide) data about serious unexpected adverse reactions/experiences, medication errors and any suspected transmission of an infectious agent through the medicinal products by marketing authorisation holders (MAHs) from direct reports and literature.

An important difference between the systems is that in the EU the MAHs have to report *all* serious adverse reactions (worldwide) as 15-day reports and in the future in addition all non-serious adverse reactions (occurring in the EU) as ICSRs within 60 days. In the USA the non-serious adverse reactions/experiences are part of the periodic adverse drug experience reports.

Healthcare professionals and patients are strongly encouraged to report *all* adverse reactions to the authorities. In accordance with the ICH E2A guideline [6], the definition of an adverse reaction implies at least a reasonable possibility of a causal relationship between a suspected medicinal product and an adverse event. An adverse reaction, in contrast to an adverse event, is characterised by the fact that a causal relationship between a medicinal product and an occurrence is suspected. If an event is spontaneously reported, even if the relationship is unknown or unstated, it meets the definition of an adverse reaction/experience (see Sect. 1.2.2).

- Therefore, all spontaneous reports notified by healthcare professionals, patients or consumers are considered suspected adverse reactions ('implied causality'), since they convey the suspicions of the primary sources, unless the reporters specifically state that they believe the events to be unrelated or that a causal relationship can be excluded.

The European Medicine Agency (EMA) and the National Competent Authorities (NCA) in the EU and the Food and Drug Administration (FDA) in the USA are empowered to impose certain obligations on authorised medicinal products, to ensure the appropriate changes to medicinal product's labelling and to conduct post-authorisation safety studies, when new safety information makes them necessary. In addition authorities can impose special risk management programmes, called risk evaluation and mitigation strategies (REMS) in the USA or Risk Management Plans in the EU [19].

1.4 Pharmacovigilance: Limitations of Clinical Trials

Randomised controlled trials normally do not have adverse events as primary endpoint. To obtain a balanced assessment of interventions (in medicine), an analysis of both benefits and harms is mandatory. In most clinical trials the study design aims at the efficacy or effectiveness of a new medicinal product or therapeutic intervention. The result of such trials is that real safety of the medicinal product/intervention used in routine work is often unknown. Also for a realistic evaluation of the risk-benefit ratio in clinical trials or statistical evaluations of post-authorisation data, a comparison between the number needed to harm versus number needed to treat would be of interest. This would show if 'common, mild, symptomatic adverse effects can affect concordance with the therapy and quality of patients' lives' [20].

In a database search from January 2008 to April 2011 for systematic reviews with adverse events as the main outcome of 4,644 systemic reviews, only 309 were selected, reporting primarily assessing harms. Systematic reviews of primary studies quite often show a poor reporting of harms data by failing to report on harms or doing so inadequately. The authors stated that 'systematic reviews with a primary objective to assess harms represent fewer than 10 % of all systematic reviews published yearly' [21]. Also the classification of adverse events in clinical trials has to follow a precise flow chart. A patient might experience 'something' in a trial, which might be recorded or not. The investigator then has to interpret this event. His information has to be coded, using a medical dictionary. In 1994 the pharmaceutical industry and regulatory authorities agreed that MedDRA (Medical Dictionary for Regulatory Activities) should be used for coding of any event. Nevertheless, different coding systems were used by pharmaceutical companies and even authorities. Depending on which dictionary is used for the coding and the interpretation of the event within the coding system, each event can be coded as several different terms, which will influence the weight of the event. Each of these different coding steps means a decision which may influence the overall impression of harms [22]. The number of published systemic reviews is increasing steadily and most of them (73.1 %) report on some aspects of harm. The results of such systemic reviews depend on data collection via databases and the use of adequate templates for the evaluation of the data. There are obvious differences between evaluating persons due to different coding systems of diagnoses. In one study comparing the interobserver variation, 12 % of the codes were evaluated differently by two codes. Another bias might be the different way of documentation of adverse events, direct contact between patient and investigator, data from medical records or laboratory results, and use of different dictionaries [23].

1.5 Pharmacovigilance: Basic Problems

On the website of the Cochrane Adverse Effects Methods Group (established in 2007), which advises the Cochrane Collaboration on how the validity and precision of systematic reviews can be improved (http://aemg.cochrane.org), the main purposes of pharmacovigilance systems are defined:

- To raise awareness of the adverse effects of interventions and to promote the inclusion of adverse effects data in Cochrane reviews
- To spread and deepen understanding of the principles, involved in assessing adverse effects
- To provide methodological guidance of specific aspects of evaluating adverse effects

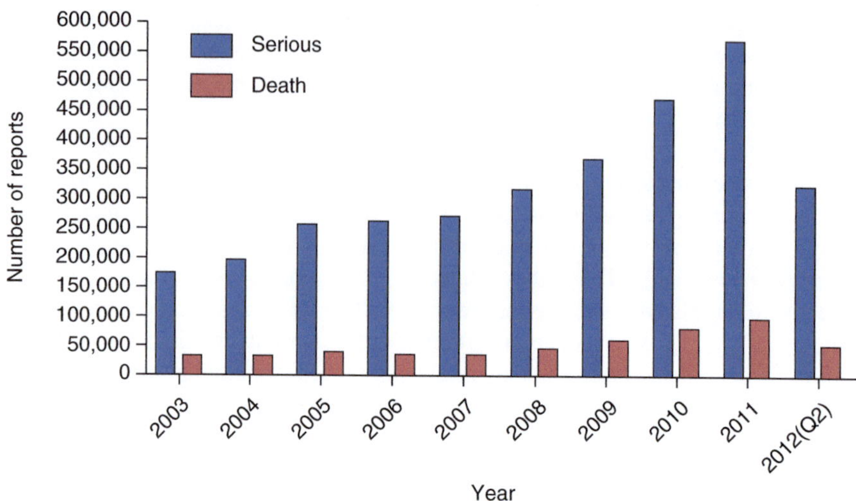

Fig. 1.3 Patient outcome(s) for reports in FAERS since the year 2003 until the second quarter of 2012. Serious events include death, hospitalisation, life-threatening, disability, congenital anomaly and/or other serious outcome [24]

To identify areas of methodological uncertainty, the fundamental statement of the Cochrane Adverse Effects Methods Group is that every healthcare intervention carries some risk of harm; the knowledge about this has to be included in the decision about the medication used for an individual patient.

The FDA is running AERS/FAERS since 1968 [24]. The number of reports is increasing steadily (Figs. 1.3 and 1.4). Same trend was observed by the German authority (Fig. 1.5).

'To date FAERS contains approximately 5 million reports and currently receives 500,000 reports per year' [26]. The FAERS is used by the FDA for the evaluation of new safety concerns and of the manufacturer's compliance to reporting regulations [22].

The EU has implemented EudraVigilance. This is a data-processing network and management system for reporting and evaluating suspected adverse reactions during development and following the marketing authorisation of medicinal products in the European Economic Area (EEA). The first operating version was launched in December 2001. In the 2013 Annual Report on EudraVigilance for the European Parliament, the Council and the Commission (reporting period, 1 January to 31 December 2013) contains an overview about the total number of reports in the database (Fig. 1.6).

Important limitations of such reporting systems:

- Many reports do not contain the information if the event was due to a specific medicinal product, especially in multi-morbidity and co-administration of multiple drugs in parallel (cross-reaction between different medicinal products?)
- In many reports not enough details for proper evaluation of a reported event.
- Very probably high numbers of adverse events that may occur from a specific product are not reported to the authorities.

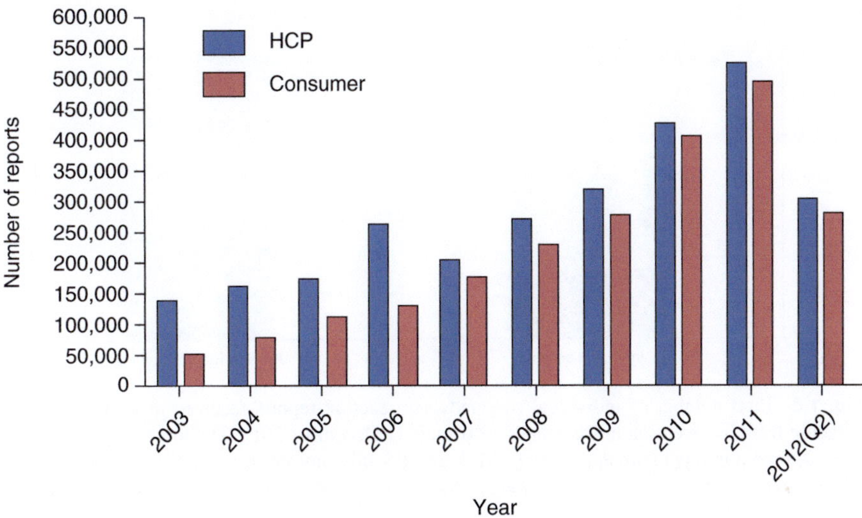

Fig. 1.4 Number of reports in FAERS by the type of reporters (healthcare professionals (HPC) and consumers) since the year 2003 until the second quarter of 2012 [24]

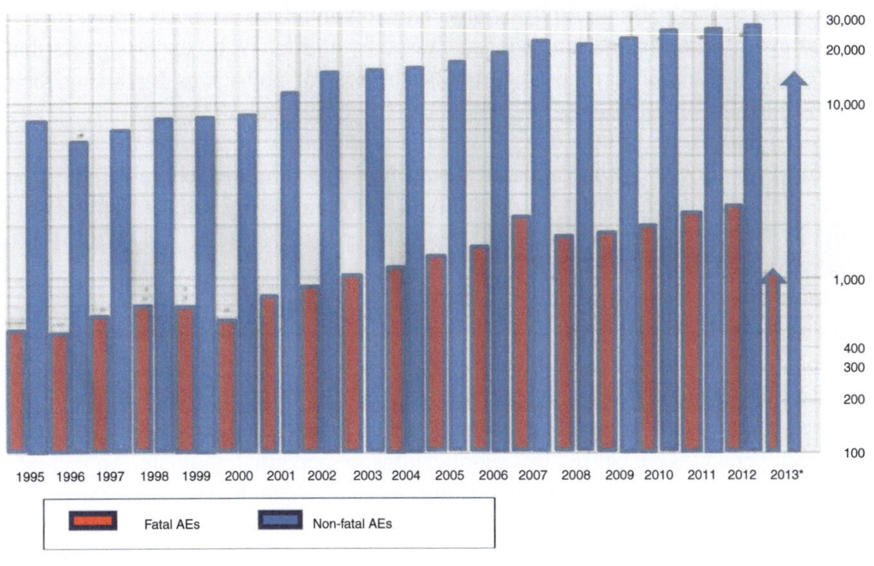

Fig. 1.5 Number of the PSURs data since the year 1995 until the second quarter of 2013 [25]

Nevertheless, if any association between a specific risk with a medicinal product becomes obvious, the above-mentioned PV activities are possible to improve the safety of the medicinal product. The essential basis for these activities is that observed adverse reactions are reported adequately by doctors and patients.

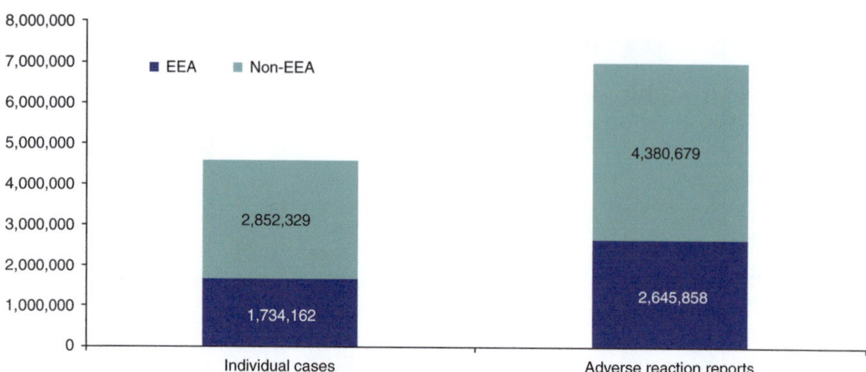

Fig. 1.6 Total number of individual cases/adverse reaction reports received in EudraVigilance database from its inception in December 2001 until 31 December 2013. The increasing number of reports, shown in this figure and Figs. 1.3, 1.4, and 1.5, does not mean per se that the incidence of adverse events is really increasing, as long as the absolute number of interventions is not known

Underreporting of adverse reactions is very common in all countries running a pharmacovigilance system. In countries participating in the WHO Drug Monitoring Program, authorities receive about 200 reports per one million inhabitants, annually from approximately 10 % of physicians. This low number of reports delays signal detection and underestimation of risks, caused by a drug. WHO experts guess that the reason for this underreporting may be the fear of physicians for losing their competence in the community or to be put at risk of litigation [15].

Other reasons might include confusion in terminology, belief that the observed reaction is already well known, medical staff time pressure or unavailable reporting forms. In a prospective study in the USA of 3,000 randomly selected physicians, only 57 % were aware of an adverse reaction reporting system, and of the 14 % observing an adverse reaction, only 0.7 % reported the occurrence [27].

Several studies reporting adverse medicinal product reactions in different institutions and countries were analysed. A few of these reviews about adverse medicinal product reactions, and events following pharmaceutical and or radiopharmaceutical interventions, will be discussed.

In a sample of 30,195 hospitalised patients, 1,133 adverse events were identified. Nineteen percent were caused by complications to medicinal products. An increasing age-related risk was observed. Patients over 64 years had adverse medicinal product reactions at a rate more than double the rate of patients ≤ 45 years [28].

In a retrospective analysis of adverse reactions and the number of really reported events, collected in an acute hospital medical setting for a period of 3 years, the data were evaluated. Following the guideline for reporting of adverse medicinal product reactions of the Committee on Safety of Medicines (CSM) in the UK, of about 23 reports per 1,000 admissions, 477 reports should have been sent. In 74.8 % ($n=357$) of these cases ($n=477$), the confirmed reaction caused admission to the hospital, but only 31 (6.5 %) of 477 potential reports were sent to the CSM [29]. In general practice, the rate of reports is only about 14 % of all suspected adverse reactions, but still greater than the reporting from hospitals. Reporting of adverse drug reactions 'is vital for the identification of previously unknown ADRs. The data are also used to assess the risk/benefit profile of both new and established drugs' [30].

The evaluation of data of the US National Centre for Health Statistics, collecting information on patient visits to outpatient clinics and emergency departments, 4,335,990 adverse drug event-related visits were counted annually with an increasing incidence from 9.0 to 17.0 per 1,000 persons between 1995 and 2005. The main risk factor in the patient groups for adverse event-related healthcare visits were patient age and polypharmacy. The proportion of outpatient visits was 6 % taking $\geq$5 medications and 14 % taking three to four medications in 1995 and in 2005 16 % vs. 17 %, respectively. These data show that the number of patients taking $\geq$5 medications more than doubled between 1995 and 2005. This will not only influence the increasing incidence of adverse drug events/experiences but also the number of drug interactions [31].

In children, a larger number of healthcare visits with an age-specific variation in the incidence of adverse events were observed. The population rate of adverse events/experiences was 13.2 visits per 1,000 children between 0 and 4 years; 4.5/1,000 between 5 and 9 years; 5.2/1,000 between 10 and 14 years; and 8.2/1,000 between 15 and 18 years. In this study, the definition of adverse events/experiences in children was different from that in adults. An adverse reaction to a medicinal product in children was defined by the authors as:

- Allergic reaction or nausea
- Dosing error or elevated drug levels with proper use of medication
- Injuries due to medication-induced dizziness [32]

In a meta-analysis of prospective trials about the incidence of adverse reactions to medicinal products in hospitalised patients, the overall incidence of adverse drug reaction was 6.7 % and for fatal events 0.32 %. From these data it has been estimated that in 1994 in US hospitals >100,000 patients died from adverse reactions to medicinal products. Probably many of these could have survived through an efficient reporting system and appropriate and current consequences [33].

In a 2-year study, 21,298 reported adverse reactions were linked to a total annual estimate of 701,547 individuals treated in emergency departments (2.4 individuals per 1,000 population). 3,487 (16 %) of the reported adverse reactions required hospitalisation. The demographic development of the population needs more attention. In 2005 about 12 % of the US population was $\geq$65 years of age, and this age group accounted for one quarter of adverse medicinal product events and 50 % needed hospitalisation [34]. This age group will increase in the near future. The data highlights the importance of an effective adverse drug reaction reporting system with surveillance of polypharmacy and drug interactions.

1.6   Radionuclide Therapy of Inflammatory Joint Diseases

One main part of this book deals with radionuclide therapy of inflammatory joint diseases. Therefore, some additional remarks about adverse reactions in nuclear medicine should be made. Especially because 'in the public arena, nuclear medicine has struggled with the widely held perception of the risk associated with radiation exposure… In the media and in public debate, and even among medical professionals, this risk is associated with other diagnostic and therapeutic interventions, obviously due to the confusion with the risks associated with nuclear power plants and nuclear weapons' [35].

Radiopharmaceuticals are used for diagnostic procedures to observe or quantify biochemical or physiological processes. This allows the visualisation of organ blood supply and/or function. The amount of radiopharmaceutical agents administered to an individual patient is usually in the microgram range and typically administered only once per study. This means that these radioactive pharmaceuticals are very rarely noxious.

In the USA, human research involving radioactive drugs has to be performed under strict rules of the Food and Drug Administration (FDA) or the Radioactive Drug Research Committee (RDRC). Similar regulations are true for EMA and many other national authorities. In a retrospective study from 1975 to 2004, the review of RDRC files dating back to 2001, no adverse reactions due to radiopharmaceutical agents in relation with medicinal products were found in human subjects [36]. Most radiopharmaceuticals do not have a pharmacological effect. Nevertheless, radiopharmaceutical agents, used in diagnostic procedures, are causing adverse reaction, but very rarely.

A comparison of adverse reactions in other diagnostic and therapeutic procedures and nuclear medicine is complicated again by different definitions of adverse reactions in both areas. In 1996 the Pharmacopoeia Committee of the Society of Nuclear Medicine (SNM) proposed the following:

Operational definition of an adverse reaction to radiopharmaceuticals:

1. 'The reaction is a noxious and unintended clinical manifestation (signs, symptoms, laboratory data abnormalities) following the administration of a radiopharmaceutical or nonradioactive adjunct pharmaceutical.
2. The reaction is not one anticipated from the known pharmacologic action of the nonradioactive pharmaceutical.
3. The reaction is not the result of an overdose (which is a misadministration).
4. The reaction is not the result of an injury caused by poor injection technique.
5. The reaction is not due to deterministic effects of therapeutic radiation (e.g. myelosuppression).
6. The definition excludes altered bio-distribution which causes no signs, symptoms or laboratory abnormalities.'

Using this definition, the published prevalence of adverse reactions to radiopharmaceuticals ranges between 0.3 and 33/100,000 administrations. This wide range is due to the widely unknown exact total number of administrations. The Pharmacopoeia

Committee of the Society of Nuclear Medicine runs a 5-year prospective study, collecting data from 18 collaborating institutes about administered radiopharmaceutical doses and adverse reactions to the radiopharmaceuticals as well as to nonradioactive pharmaceuticals used in nuclear medicine interventions (e.g. contrast media, dipyridamole, glucagon). The prevalence of adverse reactions was 2.3/100,000 administrations to radiopharmaceuticals and 5.9/100,000 to nonradioactive pharmaceuticals [37].

In another prospective survey, performed in 17 European nuclear medicine institutions, a total of 71,046 administrations of radiopharmaceuticals and 18 adverse events were reported, including 2 after radioiodine therapy. Five of the 18 adverse events were of vasovagal nature; 8 of the remaining 13 cases were classified as possibly or probably medicinal product related. Thus, the range of prevalence was between 25 (18 cases) and 11 (8 cases) per 100,000 administrations [38].

The increasing number of patients treated with multiple medications was mentioned above. This is relevant for the interpretation of 'unintended effect of a radiopharmaceutical product, occurring at doses normally used by a patient, which is related to the pharmacokinetic properties of the medicinal product'. Using radiopharmaceuticals following biochemical or physiological procedures, the biodistribution and pharmacokinetics may be altered by a variety of co-medications [30, 39, 40]. The result of such an interaction of different medicinal product may be an over- or underestimation of organ's function or disease. Therefore, changing of bio-distribution should be reported. The real number of adverse reactions in relation to medicinal product in publications and reporting systems is underestimated, but an estimate of the real number of interactions between medicinal products and radiopharmaceutical agents is totally unknown. Registration of false-positive or false-negative results due to an interaction of medicinal products in nuclear medicine, as side effect, following the definition of the WHO, is mandatory to avoid over- or under-therapy.

A Japanese group brought forward another interesting fact, influencing results of diagnostic or therapeutic procedures. Besides adverse medicinal product reactions, the authors evaluated also defect products from 1,277,907 radiopharmaceutical quality controls and administrations. Sixteen cases of adverse medicinal product reactions and eight cases of defect products were reported. The incidence of adverse medicinal product reactions was 1.3 and of defect products 0.6 per 100,000 cases, respectively [41].

Silberstein recently published data about the prevalence of adverse events to radiopharmaceuticals from 2007 to 2011 and observed a decreasing incidence of reported AEs of 3.2 to 1.6 AEs/100,000 doses. In data we could evaluate from national authorities, this is quite different, but not significantly, from country to country [42].

The quality of reports is critical for appropriate evaluation of the relationship between a medicinal product and adverse reactions. Also for the calculation of the overall incidence of an adverse event, the number of the published AEs has to be related to the number of treated patients. Although 30 serious events were listed in the PSURs of 2 companies distributing radionuclides for nuclear medicine treatment of inflammatory joint diseases (Table 1.1), 22 of them were taken from a

Table 1.1 Periodic safety update report data for the radionuclides used for radiosynovectomy

Nuclide, distributor, time period	Treated joints (n)[a]	Serious AEs (n)	Non-serious AEs (n)	Symptoms (serious AEs)
Yttrium-90citrate 1.1.1990–31.7.2011	~347,000	13 (+19[b])	11	8× bacterial infection 1× pain, immobilisation 1× anaphylactic shock 1× neurologic symptoms (off-label use for hip) 1× pulmonary embolism 1× skin necrosis (off-label use (ankle)
Yttrium-90 silicate 1.6.1994–31.8.2003	~70,000	3	2	1× anaphylactic shock 2× fever with hospitalisation
186-Rhenium sulphide 1.1.1990–21.7.2010	~200,000	13 (+ 3[b])	19	10× bacterial infection (6× same vial, same institute) 2× overdosage 1× necrosis (off-label use finger joint)
169-Erbium citrate 1.1.1990–21.7.2010	~284,000	1	10	1× immobilisation (off-label use)
Total	**~901,000**	**30 (+22[c])**	**42**	

Adapted from Fischer and Brinker [43]

[a]Number of treated joints were calculated from the amount of distributed activity

[b]Reported serious adverse events [44] was listed in the PSURs after publication, but the data of the publication were collected over a time period of 12 years. Further details are discussed in Chap. 9

[c]Symptoms of these AEs: 17× osteonecrosis, 3× infection, 2× osteonecrosis and bacterial infection

publication [44]. Few case reports were published in the annual European system for reporting reactions and defects of radiopharmaceuticals from 1994 to 2001. Case reports are quite often incomplete and the publication delay also means a delay of the registration of an adverse reaction. In the hierarchy of evidence, analytical studies are higher than case reports, but these provide more actual information about new and more previously adverse reactions/events. A better way would be to report immediately the event to the authorities and publish it later, mentioning the former report in the publication to avoid double counting. This was mentioned already above [14]. Anyway, case reports are useful to raise hypotheses about adverse reactions and events which might be studied in controlled trials [45]. The PSURs have to list such published adverse events also, without knowing detailed numbers of interventions with the medicinal product which may have caused an adverse reaction. Depending on the specificity of safety questions, the widest possible range of sources for information would be helpful finding relevant data on safety [51]. But authorisation holders would need for these reports (FAERS, PSURs) adequate information about medicinal product utilisation (determinator). These data are commonly only taken from sales data, which are not congruent with usage levels. The number of adverse reactions (nominator) is also incorrect as it is depending on reporting bias [46].

Many regulatory authorities and pharmaceutical companies are using their own signal detection algorithms (SDA), which are quite often not comparable. Therefore, published results of different authorities and pharmaceutical companies might be inconsistent [26]. For the evaluation of risk-benefit profiles of any drug, special assessment techniques are needed for development of an algorithm to get comparable safety and benefit profiles for pharmaceuticals products. The lack of standardised and validated quantitative methodology limits the outcome of explicit, consistent and transparent results of different regulatory authorities and sponsors of medicinal products [47].

Conclusion

In an editorial about 'Adverse events in randomized trials: neglected, restricted, distorted, and silenced', the author stated that 'many trials do not report harms or report them in a fragmented or suboptimal way' [48]. Raising the awareness of adverse events or reactions to medicinal products will probably result in different rates of case reporting, depending on increasing or decreasing interventions. For the calculation of the incidence of adverse reactions, the knowledge of the number is mandatory to evaluate the risk-benefit balance of an intervention. Otherwise the data may lead to an erroneous conclusion.

Another bias in official publication by authorities or pharmaceutical companies occurs when regulatory authorities and pharmaceutical companies use their own signal detection algorithms which are quite often not comparable. Therefore, the results of these publications are inconsistent. To improve this standardisation of reporting systems of national and international regulatory authorities as well as of analytic practices and terminology also for manufacturers of medicinal products, researchers and authors are needed, to monitor safety concern and risks associated with these products [26, 49]. It is well known and even stated in the EMA guideline on good pharmacovigilance practices that risk minimisation measures are 'an evolving area of medical science with no universally agreed standards and approaches' [13].

Following the aims of pharmacovigilance for enhancement of patient care and safety in relation to the administration of medicines and in support of public health programmes by providing reliable information for the effective assessment of the risk-benefit profile of medicinal products further, standardisation of reporting systems, archiving and publication rules are needed.

Cochrane Adverse Event Method Group recommended to raise awareness of adverse events. In publications of different parts of the world, authors complain low reporting and low physicians' awareness of pharmacovigilance systems and necessity of training programmes. The American College of Physicians recommended in 2009 to strengthen the efforts to improve education of health professionals on how and when to report adverse reactions/events [51]. Several authors from different parts of the world [52–55] observed in their countries a lack of interest in pharmacovigilance and education in reporting systems. But education is the cornerstone of a functioning system. The evaluation of teaching programmes in the UK showed that only half of the respondents provided undergraduate students with a guide for reporting adverse reactions. In the USA, Centers for Education and Research in Therapeutics (CERTS) should educate healthcare professionals in pharmacovigilance systems, how to recognise and to report adverse reaction to minimise patient's risk. In 1997 six centres started with an annual budget of about $ 5.9 million. In 2010/2011 the number of CERTS had increased up to 14, but in 2012 in the annual report of CERTS only again 6 centres were listed (www.certs.hhs.gov). It is worth to compare the yearly budget of CERTS with the expenses of Medicare for medicinal product in 2006 ($ 70 billion), of the pharmaceutical industry on research and development (>$30 billion) and promotion ($ >15 billion) [56].

It is likely that the situation of institutes dealing with pharmacovigilance training might be the same in EU. But in the EU, as concordant with many other countries, each pharmaceutical company has to have a qualified person, responsible for the internal pharmacovigilance system, and has also to train the staff. This is controlled by inspections of the authorities. To improve low reporting and awareness of pharmacovigilance systems, this topic should become part of continuing medical education for physicians. Each medical institution and department should make training of their staff regarding pharmacovigilance activities an essential part of their quality management system. More complicated is the training of consumers, because they show low knowledge about available reporting systems and the reports depend on special situations. In Australia, consumers' reporting was 5.7 % of known adverse events between 2003 and 2009, 9.8 % in 2009 because of a H1N1 influenza and 3 % in 2011 [52]. To improve these deficits, pharmacovigilance should become part of continuing medical education, standard operating procedures in all medical institutes and practices guiding training of the medical staff.

Errors in therapy with medicines may lead to serious adverse reactions. As a result, studies show that about 5.7 % of hospitalised patients are affected by a serious adverse reaction and that about 4.8 % of hospital admissions are due to serious adverse reactions. This percentage is significantly higher for older patients with about 10–15 %. An analysis indicates that 31–58 % of these errors are mistakes in dosing. Particularly overdoses are observed, of which 30–40 % to a lack of dose adjustment in patients suffering from renal insufficiency and another 19 % are due to a failure to adapt the dose to the patient's weight. The non-observance of allergies and of therapeutically relevant interactions and contraindications leads to avoidable adverse reactions, because medicinal products are prescribed that are unsuitable for the patient [57].

As many as 1.5 million Americans are injured or killed each year by inappropriate use (including errors and misuse) of FDA-regulated drugs [18], and fatal adverse reactions may be number 4–6 of the leading causes of death in the USA. Some of the deficits in the pharmacovigilance systems do not only cause harm to patients but are also important for the national economy. If at least one in seven patient episodes is complicated by an adverse reaction, nearly 2 % of bed days in the UK were due to an ADR. The authors estimated roughly annual ADR costs of approximately £ 5,000 per hospital bed [58].

Individual and systemic strategies to avoid medication errors are available. It is important to implement a safety culture and to bring together the therapeutic expertise and cooperation between the partners in healthcare, in the interest and well-being of patients.

References

1. WHO. The importance of pharmacovigilance, safety monitoring of medicinal products. World Health Organisation, Geneva 2002.
2. The world medicines situation 2001 – pharmacovigilance and safety of medicines. World Health Organisation, Geneva 2011.
3. FDA Adverse Event Reporting System (FAERS) (http://www.fda.gov). Glossary of terms used in pharmacovigilance. Glossary11.doc Mar 2011.
4. Meyboom RHB, Lindquist M, Egberts ACG. An ABC of drug-related problems. Drug Saf. 2000;22(6):415–28.
5. ICH. E2D guideline post-approval safety data management. Definitions and standards for expedited reporting. Oct 1994. International conferences on harmonisation of technical requirements for registration of pharmaceuticals for human use. http://www.ich.org.
6. ICH. E2D guideline clinical safety data management: definitions and standards for expedited reporting. Oct 1994. International conferences on harmonisation of technical requirements for registration of pharmaceuticals for human use. http://www.ich.org.
7. Directive 2001/83/EC on the Community code related to medicinal products for human use. REGULATION (EC) No 726/2004 of the EUROPEAN PARLIAMENT and of the COUNCIL of 31 March 2004, laying down community procedures for the authorisation and supervision of medicinal products for human and veterinary use and establishing a European Medicines Agency, as amended, i. e. Regulation (EU) 1235/2010 of the European Parliament and of the Council of December 15, 2010 amending, as regards pharmacovigilance of medicinal products for human use, Regulation (EC) N0 726/2004 laying down Community procedures for the authorisation and supervision of medicinal products for human and veterinary use and establishing a European Medicines Agency, and Regulation (EC) No 1394/2007 on advanced therapy medicinal products. European Commission's Implementing Regulation (EU) No 520/2012 of 19 June 2012 on the performance of pharmacovigilance activities provided for in Regulation (EC) No 726/2004 of the European Parliament and of the Council and Directive 2001/83/EC of the European Parliament and of the Council, Official Journal of the European Union, 20.6.2012, L 159/5.
8. EMA/876333/2011. Rev.3* guideline on good pharmacovigilance practices (GVP) Annex I-definitions(Rev.3.) European medicines agency and heads of medicines agencies 2014.
9. EMA/873138/2011. Guideline on good pharmacovigilance practices (GVP) module VI – management and reporting of adverse reactions to medicinal products (Rev 1).
10. EMA guideline on good pharmacovigilance practicies (GVP) module IX-signal management. European medicines agency and heads of medicines agencies 2014.
11. ICH. E2B guideline: periodic benefit-risk evaluation report. Mar 2014. International conferences on harmonisation of technical requirements for registration of pharmaceuticals for human use. http://www.ich.org.
12. Report of the Council for International Organisations of Medical Sciences Working group VIII "practical aspects of signal detection in pharmacovigilance". Geneva: CIOMS; 2010.
13. EMA guideline on good pharmacovigilance practicies (GVP) module XVI, risk minimisation measures: selection and effectiveness indicators. (Rev. 1.) European medicines agency and heads of of medicines agencies 2014.
14. Sickmüller B, Thurisch B, Kaszkin-Bettag M. Letter to the editor – proposal for publishing of case reports of adverse drug reactions to authorities by physicians. Glob Adv Health Med. 2013. doi:10.7453/gahmj.2013.007.

15. ICH. E2B guideline on clinical safety data management: data elements for transmission of individual case safety reports. Feb 2001. International conferences on harmonisation of technical requirements for registration of pharmaceuticals for human use. http://www.ich.org.
16. U.S. Department of Health and Human Services. Guidance for industry – good pharmacovigilance practices and pharmacovigilance assessment. (J:/!Guidanc/63590=CC.doc). Mar 2005.
17. CRF- Code of Federal Regulations Title 21; Part 314 applications for FDA approval to market new drugs. http://www.accessdata.fda.gov.
18. Advances in FDA's safety program for marketed drugs, establishing premarket safety review and marketed drug safety as equal priorities at FDA's center for drug evaluation and research, drug safety center for drug evaluation and research, U.S. Food and Drug Administration U.S. Health and Human Services Report; April 2012.
19. Sheikholeslam AS. Comparison of EU-Pharmacovigilance system master file (PSMF) with US system. Wissenschaftliche Prüfungsarbeit zur Erlangung des Titels "Master of Drug Regulatory Affairs". Bonn; 2013.
20. Aronson JK, Derry S, Loke YK. Adverse drug reactions: keeping up to date. Fundam Clin Pharmacol. 2002;16:49–56.
21. Zorzela L, Golder S, Liu Y, et al. Quality of reporting in systematic reviews of adverse events: systematic review. BMJ. 2014;348:f7668. doi:10.1136/bmj.f7668.
22. Schroll JB, Maund E, Gøtzsche PC. Challenges in coding adverse events in clinical trials: a systematic review. PLoS One. 2012;7:e41174. doi:10.1371/journal.pone.0041174.
23. Moher D, Tetzlaff J, Tricco AC, et al. Epidemiology and reporting characteristics of systemic reviews. PLoS Med. 2007;4:447–55.
24. FDA Adverse Events Reports. http://www.fda.gov.
25. Pharmakovigilanz. 2014 http://www.BfArM.
26. Harpaz R, DuMouchel W, LePendu P, et al. Performance of pharmacovigilance signal detection algorithms for FDA adverse event reporting system. Clin Pharmacol Ther. 2013;93. doi:10.1038/clpt.213.24.
27. Rogers AS, Israel E, Smith CR, et al. Physician knowledge, attitudes and behavior related to reporting adverse drug events. Arch Intern Med. 1988;148:1596–600.
28. Leape LL, Brennan TA, Laird N, et al. The nature of adverse events in hospitalized patients. Results of the Harvard Medical Practice Study II. N Engl J Med. 1991;324:377–84.
29. Heeley E, Riley J, et al. Prescription-event monitoring and reporting of adverse drug reactions. Lancet. 2001;358:1872–3.
30. Smith CC, Bennett PM, Pearce HM, et al. Adverse drug reactions in a hospital general medical meriting notification to the Committee of Safety of Medicines. Br J Clin Pharmacol. 1996;42:423–9.
31. Bourgeois FT, Shannon MW, Valim C, Mandl KD. Adverse drug events in the outpatient setting: an 11-year national analysis. Pharmacoepidemiol Drug Saf. 2010;19:901–10. 1.
32. Bourgeois FT, Mandl KD, Valim C, Shannon MW. Pediatric adverse drug events in the outpatient setting: an 11-year national analysis. Pediatrics. 2009;124:744–50.
33. Lazarou J, Pomeranz BH, Corey PN. Incidence of adverse drug reactions in hospitalised patients. A meta-analysis of prospective studies. JAMA. 1998;279:1200–5.
34. Budnitz DS, Pollock DA, Weidenbach KN, et al. National surveillance of emergency department visits for outpatient adverse drug events. JAMA. 2006;296:1858–66.
35. Hesse B, Vinberg N, Berthelsen AK, Ballinger JR. Adverse events in nuclear medicine – cause for concern? Eur J Nucl Med Mol Imaging. 2012;39:782–5.
36. Suleiman OH, Fejka R, Houn F, Walsh M. The radioactive drug research committee: background and retrospective study of reported research data (1975–2004). J Nucl Med. 2006;47:1220–6.

37. Silberstein EB, Ryan J. Prevalence of adverse reactions in nuclear medicine. J Nucl Med 1996;37:185–92. Hesslewood SR, Keeling DH, Radiopharmacy committee of EANM. Frequency of adverse reactions to radiopharmaceuticals in Europe. Eur J Nucl Med. 1997;24:1179–82.

38. Hesslewood SR, Keeling DH. Radiopharmacy Committee of the EANM. Frequency of adverse reactions to radiopharmaceuticals in Europe. Eur J Nucl Med. 1997;24:1179–82.

39. Santos-Oliveira R. Undesirable events with radiopharmaceuticals. Tohoku J Exp Med. 2009;217:251–7.

40. Santos-Oliveira R, Smith SW, Carneiro-Leao AMA. Radiopharmaceuticals drug interactions: a critical review. An Acad Bras Cienc. 2008;80:665–75.

41. Kusakabe K, Okamura T Kassagi K, Komatani A, et al. Subcommittee for safety issues of Radiopharmaceuticals, Medical Science, and Pharmaceutical Committee, Japan Radioisotope Association. The 27th report on survey of the adverse reactions to radiopharmaceuticals (the 30th survey in 2004) Kaku Igaku. 2006;43:23–5.

42. Siberstein EB. Prevalence of adverse events to radiopharmaceuticals from 2007 to 2011. J Nucl Med. 2014;55:1308–10.

43. Fischer M, Brinker A. Legal responsibility of the nuclear medicine physician at the radiosynoviorthesis and radionuclide therapy of bone metastases. Der Nuklearmediziner. 2013;36:53–60.

44. Kisielinski K, Bremer D, Knutsen A, et al. Complications following radiosynoviorthesis in osteoarthritis and arthroplasty: osteonecrosis and intra-articular infection. Joint Bone Spine. 2010;77:252–7.

45. Hennessy S. Disproportionality analyses of spontaneous reports – editorial. Pharmacoepidem Drug Saf. 2004;13:503–4.

46. Hazel L, Shakir SAW. Under-reporting of adverse drug reactions – a systematic review. Drug Saf. 2006;29:385–96.

47. Guo JJ, Pandey S, Doyle J, et al. A review of quantitative risk – benefit methodologies for assessing drug safety and efficacy-report of the ISPOR Risk-Benefit Management Working Group. Value Health. 2010;13:657–66.

48. Ioannidis JPA. Adverse events in randomized trials. Arch Intern Med. 2009;169:1737–9.

49. Lis Y, Guo JJ, Roberts MH, et al. Comparisons of Food and Drug Administration and European Medicines Agency risk management implementation for recent pharmaceutical approvals: report of the International Society for Pharmacoeconomics and Outcomes Research Risk Benefit Management Working Group. Value Health. 2012;15:1108–18.

50. Pilkington K, Boshnakova A. Complementary medicine and safety: a systematic investigation of design and reporting of systematic reviews. Complement Ther Med. 2012;20:73–82.

51. American College of Physicians. Improving FDA regulations of prescription drugs. Policy Monograph, Philadelphia; 2009.

52. Robertson J, Newby DA, Robertson J. Low awareness of adverse drug reaction reporting systems: a consumer survey. Med J Aust. 2013;199:684–6.

53. Katamne RA, Jayawardhani. Knowledge, attitude and perception of physicians towards adverse drug reactions (ADR) reporting: a pharmacoepidemiological study. Asian J Pharm Clin Res. 2012;5:210–4.

54. Iffat W, Shakeel S, et al. Pakistani physicians' knowledge and attitude towards reporting adverse drug reactions. Afr J Pharm Pharmacol. 2014;8:379–85.

55. Hudec R, Wilton LV, Kriska M. Comments to regional problems of analgesic risk perception. Bratisl Lek Listy. 2011;12:140–2.

56. Strom BL. How the US drug safety system should be changed. JAMA. 2006;295:2072–5.

57. Schnurrer J, Frölich JC. Zur Häufigkeit und Vermeidbarkeit von tödlichen unerwünschten Arzneimittelwirkung. Internist. 2003;44:889–95.

58. Davies EC, Green CF, et al. Adverse drug reactions in hospital in-patients: a prospective analysis of patient-episodes. PLoS One. 2009;4(2):e4439. doi:10.1371/journal.pone.0004439.

Part I

Histopathology and Non-radioactive Treatment of Synovitis

The Role of Synovial Macrophages in Rheumatoid Arthritis and Osteoarthritis: Its Implications for Radiosynovectomy

Jan Bondeson

Contents

2.1 Introduction

Mononuclear phagocytes are defined as the descendants of haematopoietic stem cells that develop sequentially into monoblasts, promonocytes, monocytes and macrophages. The newly formed monocytes leave the bone marrow and enter the circulation. They later leave the bloodstream to become resident tissue macrophages; the majority migrate to the liver, while others reside in the spleen, lungs and other tissues. There are also macrophages in the pleural and peritoneal cavities. Resident tissue macrophages are usually in a resting state, but they can easily become activated by various stimuli. The macrophage surface membrane contains a great variety of specific receptors. The activated macrophage is a potent phagocyte and serves as a scavenger of live or dead microorganisms, debris and dying cells. It is also a key player in the induction and regulation of acute and chronic inflammation through its many bioactive secretory products, including cytokines, proteases, complement components and arachidonic acid metabolites (Figs. 2.1 and 2.2).

J. Bondeson, MD, PhD
Department of Rheumatology, Cardiff University, Heath Park, Cardiff CF14 4XN, UK
e-mail: BondesonJ@cf.ac.uk

© Springer International Publishing Switzerland 2015
W.U. Kampen, M. Fischer (eds.), *Local Treatment of Inflammatory Joint Diseases: Benefits and Risks*, DOI 10.1007/978-3-319-16949-1_2

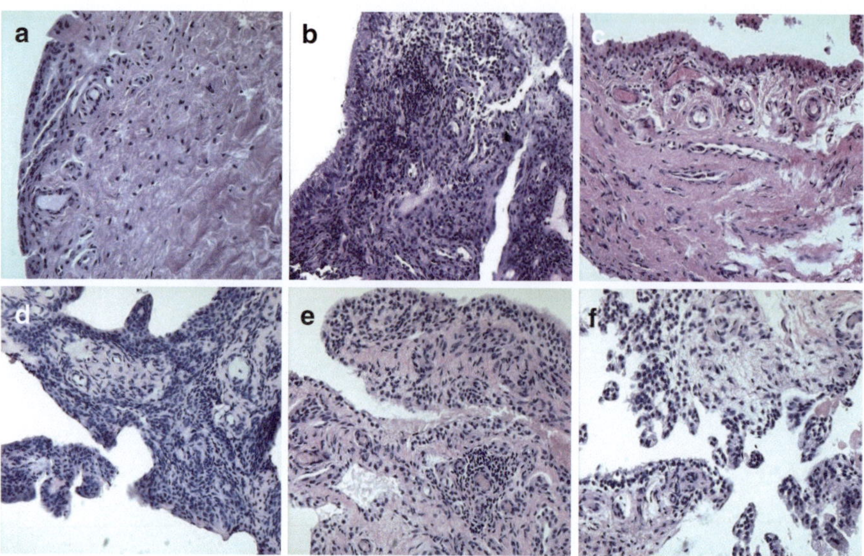

Fig. 2.1 Histology of early OA (**a**–**c**) and RA (**d**–**f**) samples, indicating thickened synovium and infiltration of inflammatory cells. The histology changes in early OA can be quite suggestive of inflammation, even resembling the changes seen in RA

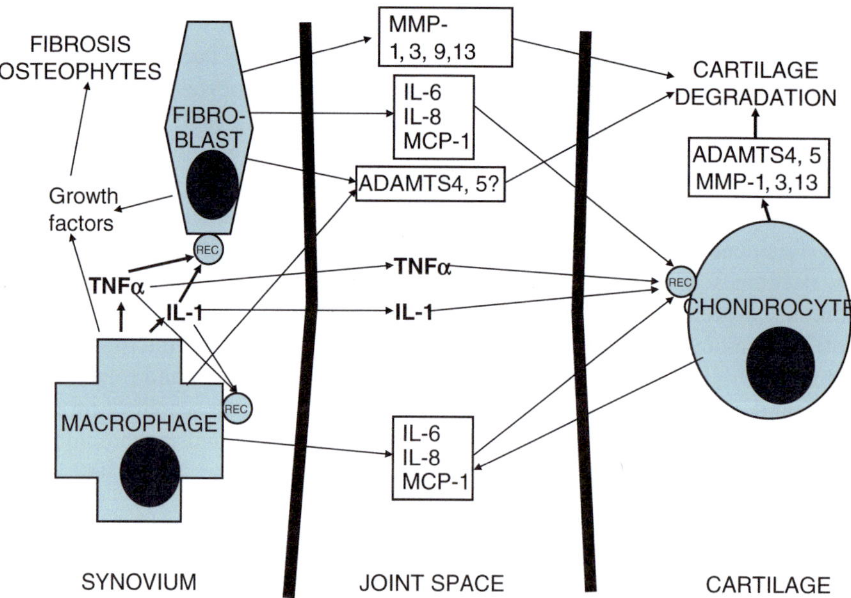

Fig. 2.2 A simplified view of cell signalling in the OA synovium and the production of inflammatory and destructive mediators

Rheumatoid arthritis (RA) is the most common of the inflammatory arthritides and a both important and treatable disease. It is characterised by intense synovial inflammation and proliferation, giving rise to cartilage destruction and bony erosions. In RA, it is today accepted that both inflammatory and destructive features of the disease are driven through synovitis. The RA synovium has a plentiful infiltrate of activated macrophages, particularly at the cartilage-pannus junction [1]. These macrophages produce tumour necrosis factor-α (TNFα), interleukin (IL)-1β and other proinflammatory cytokines. Since there is a 'cytokine cascade' with TNFα driving many of the other inflammatory mediators, this cytokine has become a key therapeutic target in RA, with several anti-TNFα biologic agents being used with considerable success [2]. Although biologics with anti-B-cell and anti-T-cell co-stimulation properties have since been introduced, as well as anti-IL6-receptor antibodies, the anti-TNFα agents remain a mainstay of RA therapy, with long-term sustained efficacy and safety.

Osteoarthritis (OA), one of the most common diseases among mammals, is characterised pathologically by focal areas of damage on articular cartilage centred on load-bearing areas, associated with formation of new bone at the joint margins and changes in subchondral bone. Given the huge economic and personal burden of OA, and the fact that this disease is the major cause for the increasing demand for joint replacements, there is urgent need for disease-modifying treatments to stop or at least slow the development and progression of OA. Various drug candidates have been brought forward, but hitherto, none of them has been clearly demonstrated to have clinical benefit in OA [3, 4]. Nor have the widely available 'nutraceuticals' glucosamine and chondroitin sulphate been demonstrated to have benefit in this disease [5].

The role of macrophages driving inflammatory and destructive pathways in RA is still controversial. Clinically, OA patients have a variable degree of synovitis, sometimes with quite aggressive large-joint arthritis with exudation. There is evidence that this synovitis is macrophage driven and that it contributes to disease progression in early stages of OA. When OA is clinically significant, disease is already well advanced, however, and clinical trials of strategies directed against macrophage-produced cytokines have not been successful. The concept of inflammatory synovitis contributing to OA pathology has attracted interest for some time [6–8], particularly the role of activated synovial macrophages in driving inflammatory and destructive pathways in the OA synovitis [9, 10], but the path from the introduction of this concept to its utilisation for the potential development of a disease-modifying anti-osteoarthritic drug remains a lengthy one.

This chapter will give an overview of some important recent findings concerning the ability of macrophages to drive inflammatory and destructive disease mechanisms in RA and OA, the role of their proinflammatory cytokines in doing so and the potential for macrophages and macrophage-produced cytokines to be used as therapeutic targets for the development of disease-modifying drugs. The role of synovial macrophages in the mechanism of action of radiosynovectomy in RA and OA will also be discussed.

2.2   The Role of Macrophages in RA

RA is a common (prevalence 1 % in Europe and the USA) and potentially debilitating inflammatory disease, recognised in Europe since the early 1800s. It mainly involves joint inflammation but also has systemic manifestations in many patients, like rheumatoid nodules, anaemia and bone marrow changes, lung fibrosis, pleuritis and pericarditis, eye disease with scleritis or episcleritis and occasionally small vessel vasculitis. Clinically, RA presents with symmetrical inflammatory arthritis involving both large and small joints, typically the wrists, metacarpophalangeal joints and proximal interphalangeal joints, as well as early symmetrical involvement of the metatarsophalangeal joints. Typically, there is visible and palpable joint swelling, caused by synovial inflammation and hypertrophy, and exudation of excess of synovial fluid. In severe early RA, there is pronounced morning stiffness, sometimes lasting for hours, and generalised weakness, malaise and low-grade fever. If RA is left untreated, there will be progressive development of joint erosions involving both cartilage and subchondral bone, as well as joint contractures leading to permanent disability. These joint erosions can be seen on plain X-rays, and early on an MRI scan, and they thus have diagnostic value. Since erosions are irreversible, causing permanent structural damage, there is a need for a swift diagnosis for the disease to be challenged with the most potent disease-modifying antirheumatic drugs (DMARDs).

The American College of Rheumatology (ACR) has established a set of seven criteria (symmetrical arthritis, hand arthritis, polyarthritis, significant morning stiffness, erosions, rheumatoid nodules and rheumatoid factor positivity) that are both useful and generally accepted. As soon as these criteria are fulfilled, the practice is to institute treatment with one of the most potent DMARDs: methotrexate, sulphasalazine or leflunomide. Therapeutic concentrations of some of the old-fashioned DMARDs, like auranofin and the antimalarials chloroquine and hydroxychloroquine, appear to have an effect on macrophage-produced proinflammatory cytokines [11], although nontoxic concentrations of methotrexate or leflunomide do not [11, 12]. The problems with these DMARDs are that they are not sufficiently potent in many patients, that they have severe and frequent side effects and that it is impossible to predict the response to a certain DMARD. Partial control of inflammation in RA does not appear to prevent joint damage in RA, and the majority of patients with active disease become disabled within 20 years. For those with active disease or extra-articular manifestations, the mortality is comparable to that of patients with three-vessel coronary arteriosclerosis or stage IV Hodgkin's disease [13, 14].

The inflamed RA synovium contains a mixed population of cells. Apart from the synovial fibroblasts, there are activated B and T cells, plasma cells, mast cells and activated macrophages. These cells have all been recruited via a neovascularisation process with associated lymphangiogenesis. In RA, the synovial lining, normally just two to three cells thick, becomes eight to ten cells thick, with infiltration of synovial fibroblasts and macrophages. The sublining area of the synovium, which normally has relatively few cells, becomes heavily infiltrated with inflammatory cells, macrophages prominent among them. This accumulation of cellular infiltrate is accompanied by neoangiogenesis, with an extensive network of newly formed blood vessels. The hypertrophied pannus invades and destroys cartilage and subchondral bone, and activated macrophages are particularly numerous at the cartilage-pannus junction. A study of synovial biopsies showed a clear correlation between macrophage activation markers and the general inflammatory activity [15]. Another study observed a correlation between macrophage numbers in the lining and sublining layers of the rheumatoid synovium and the subsequent development of erosions [16]. Macrophages expressing the cytokines IL-1α and TNFα are prominent near the cartilage-pannus junction [17]. Apart from their antigen-presenting capacity, these macrophages probably do not have a direct causal pathogenic effect in RA, but they remain key players in mediating inflammation and joint destruction in acute and chronic RA, as mediators of proinflammatory, destructive and tissue remodelling in this disease.

The RA synovial macrophages are in a highly activated state, overexpressing a number of cytokines that mediate local and systemic inflammation and tissue remodelling [1]. They also overexpress chemokines like IL-8, macrophage inflammatory protein 1 and monocyte chemoattractant protein 1, which stimulate migration of inflammatory cells and stimulate angiogenesis. Although the synovial fibroblasts are the main producers of matrix metalloproteinases (MMPs) in RA, macrophages can produce MMP-9 and MMP-12, as well as tissue inhibitor of metalloproteases 1, which attempts to control excessive tissue destruction. In RA, it is today accepted that the synovitis is mainly cytokine driven, through a disequilibrium between proinflammatory (TNFα, IL-1) and anti-inflammatory (IL-10, the IL-1 receptor antagonist, soluble TNF receptors) cytokines. These proinflammatory cytokines are largely produced by synovial macrophages. A key early observation was when cocultures of rheumatoid synovial cells were treated with neutralising anti-TNF antibodies, the production of another key proinflammatory cytokine, IL-1, practically ceased [18]. Further experiments showed that other proinflammatory cytokines, like IL-6, IL-8 and GM-CSF, were also driven by TNF in RA synovial cell cocultures [19–21]. These observations laid the foundation for the concept of macrophage-produced TNFα as the main mediator of disease, driving the other proinflammatory cytokines through occupying a key position at the apex of a cytokine cascade.

The hypothesis of TNFα as the dominant proinflammatory mediator in rheumatoid inflammation was tested in a model of murine collagen-induced arthritis, using either specific anti-TNF monoclonal antibodies or a soluble TNF receptor fused to the immunoglobulin Fc fragment, both of which potently ameliorated clinical symptoms of arthritis and prevented joint destruction [22, 23]. The first clinical trial of anti-TNF therapy in RA was begun in 1992, using the chimeric anti-TNF monoclonal antibody infliximab. This short-term open-label trial enrolled 20 patients, and although it was primarily intended to test dosing and safety, patients experienced a marked reduction in pain, stiffness and joint swelling within 24 h [24]. A subsequent multicentre, placebo-controlled, randomised double-blind study in 73 patients with active RA used a single intravenous infusion of either placebo, 1 mg/kg of infliximab, or 10 mg/kg of infliximab. An intention-to-treat analysis showed that only 2 of 24 placebo patients responded after 4 weeks, versus 11 of 25 patients treated with 1 mg/kg infliximab and 19 of 24 patients treated with 10 mg/kg infliximab. In patients receiving the higher dose, response duration was 8 weeks. There were impressive reductions in tender joint count, as well as in laboratory markers of disease activity, such as IL-6, CRP and ESR [25]. In a longer-term multicentre placebo-controlled, randomised, double-blind phase II study in 101 RA patients who had active disease in spite of methotrexate treatment, patients who received 3 or 10 mg/kg infliximab again showed excellent responses, although patients who received 1 mg/kg had a shorter duration of response. There was a clear synergy between infliximab and methotrexate in this study, indicating different mechanisms of action for these two compounds [26]. These data provided the rationale for a randomised phase III study of infliximab, the Anti-TNF Therapy of Rheumatoid Arthritis with Concomitant Methotrexate (ATTRACT) trial, a multicentre study involving 428 patients with active RA in spite of methotrexate treatment. The patients were split into five groups: one receiving placebo, the other four either 3 or 10 mg/kg infliximab at four-weekly or eight-weekly intervals. Again, benefit from infliximab was both swift and pronounced, with 60–70 % improvement in the tender joint count and normalisation of the CRP after the first infusion [27]. The medication was well tolerated, and the response was sustained until the 54-week end point of the study. In this trial, it was also possible to evaluate the development of joint damage through modified Sharp scoring of radiographs of the hands and feet. In the 88 patients treated with methotrexate and placebo, the median increase in this index was 4.0, but in the 340 patients treated with methotrexate and different regimens of infliximab, the score was unchanged. Thus, control of RA inflammation by infliximab prevented cartilage degradation and bony erosions [28].

As a consequence of the pivotal clinical studies quoted above, neutralisation of TNFα, the most important proinflammatory cytokine in the rheumatoid synovium, has become the preferred strategy to modulate macrophage function in RA. Infliximab (Remicade) is today one of the established biologics for the treatment of RA. The second anti-TNF therapeutic strategy in RA is the p75 TNF receptor Ig fusion protein etanercept (Enbrel), for which clinical studies were completed in 1998, with benefit similar to that observed with infliximab [29, 30]. The third available anti-TNF biologic was adalimumab (Humira), a fully human anti-TNFα antibody; it was followed by the PEGylated certolizumab pegol (Cimzia) and by golimumab (Simponi). All these five biologics have been widely approved for use on both sides of the Atlantic and are commercially available; there are even more anti-TNF biologics being developed, one of them the PEGylated soluble TNF receptor pegsunercept, as well as 'biosimilars' or follow-on biologics, which are likely to have an impact in the near future. Long-term data has shown that these anti-TNF biologics are both safe and effective: in the majority of patients, response is sustained over a 5-year period, or longer [31–33]. If patients are chosen wisely, and frail and elderly people avoided, along with those at risk for opportunistic infections, and careful screening for latent tuberculosis performed prior to treatment initiation, the drugs are perfectly safe even for long-term use. Indications for the anti-TNF biologics have widened from RA and Crohn's disease to encompass other forms of arthritis, such as severe or moderate psoriatic arthritis, early and severe ankylosing spondylitis and polyarticular juvenile idiopathic arthritis; some of them have plaque psoriasis and ulcerative colitis as indications, and they are undergoing clinical trials in a variety of inflammatory disorders. Regulatory authorities have been forced to 'ration' the anti-TNF biologics, and the current recommendation from the UK National Institute of Clinical Excellence is that to qualify for treatment with an anti-TNF biologic, patients must have failed two DMARDs, one of which must be methotrexate.

The development of biologic anti-TNF therapy against RA and other inflammatory diseases invigorated the search for other therapeutic targets in RA, with much money invested from the pharmaceutic industry, and some very promising results. The biologic rituximab (MabThera), an anti-CD20 antibody targeting B cells, which was previously used for B-cell lymphoma, has been proven to be safe and effective in RA. Several other anti-B-cell biologics, like ocrelizumab, ofatumumab and atacicept, are in clinical development. The humanised monoclonal antibody tocilizumab (RoActemra) that binds to membrane-bound and soluble forms of the IL-6 receptor has recently been found superior to adalimumab in monotherapy in a phase 4 trial in RA [34]. The anti-IL-6 antibody sarilumab and the anti-IL-6 receptor clazakizumab are both in clinical development. Another novel strategy concerns blocking T-cell co-stimulation via the anti-CTLA4 antibody abatacept (Orencia). There are many more antirheumatic drugs in development, both biologics and small molecules. The monoclonal antibodies secukinumab and brodalumab target the IL-17 family of cytokines. The small molecule tofacitinib (Xeljanz) is a Janus kinase (JAK) 3 inhibitor, which has been approved for the treatment of moderate to severe RA in the USA but not in the UK or in continental Europe. Baricitinib and ruxolitinib are two JAK 1/2 inhibitors in clinical development.

At the present time, making use of an anti-TNF biologic to block TNFα may well be the safest and most effective way to modulate macrophage function in RA, but much research has gone into investigating other options. For several decades, there has been a search for small-molecule inhibitors of TNFα production. Since it is known that in RA, the spontaneous production of TNFα from the synovial macrophages is NFκB dependent [35], there has been interest in inhibitors of this transcription factor, although NFκB is too ubiquitous a transcription factor for systemic inhibition to be clinically feasible. There has been interest in intra-articular administration of NFκB inhibitors, however, although this would only have a monoarticular effect [36, 37]. The phosphodiesterase 4 inhibitor apremilast (Otezla) has been reported to inhibit the spontaneous production of TNFα from RA synovial macrophages [38]. It is approved for the treatment of psoriatic arthritis in the USA but not as yet for RA. There is a good deal of recent literature on macrophages in RA, and the potential to induce macrophage apoptosis, to deplete synovial macrophages, or to change the macrophage polarisation from a M1 (classical, inflammatory) to M2 (alternative, anti-inflammatory) [39–41]. It has been demonstrated that RA synovial lining macrophages express folate receptor-β, and there has been an interest in targeting this to administer either folate antagonists [42] or an immunotoxin reducing the number of macrophages and inducing benefit in an animal model of arthritis [43].

2.3 The Role of Macrophages in OA

Clinically, RA and OA are usually easy to differentiate. In RA, X-rays of affected joints show erosions and periarticular osteoporosis, whereas in OA, they show reduction of joint space as a sign of cartilage degradation and, in later stages of the disease, bony sclerosis and osteophytes. The joint pattern differs, with early RA affecting the proximal interphalangeal, metacarpophalangeal and metatarsophalangeal joints and OA usually affecting the large joints, like the hips and knees, and also the distal interphalangeal joints. RA patients have an elevated erythrocyte sedimentation rate and C-reactive protein; the vast majority of OA patients do not. In RA patients, synovitis is a major feature of the disease, causing joint swelling and exudation and driving cartilage degradation and the formation of pannus and erosive changes. In OA, there is much less joint swelling and exudation and no pannus or erosions. But still, many OA patients have a variable degree of synovitis. Some of them may develop quite aggressive inflammatory OA of the knee or hip joint, sometimes with marked exudation, which can be helped by arthrocentesis and injection of local steroids. Synovial inflammation is likely to contribute to disease progression in OA, as judged by the correlation between biological markers of inflammation and the progression of structural changes in OA [44, 45]. Histologically, the OA synovium shows hyperplasia with an increased number of lining cells and a mixed inflammatory infiltrate mainly consisting of macrophages [46]. Synovial biopsies from patients with early inflammatory OA may even resemble RA biopsies morphologically, although the percentage of macrophages is lower (1–3 % as compared with 5–20 %) and the percentages of T and B cells much lower [47–49]. The marked differences in cell percentages in the inflammatory infiltrate between RA and OA would speak in favour of differences also in the cytokine interdependence in these two diseases. For example, the great scarcity of T cells in the OA synovium would tend to rule them (and their cytokines) out as potential drivers of synovitis in this disease. The synovial fluid of patients with active RA synovitis and effusion contains numerous polymorphonuclear leucocytes, something that is not the case in OA, another indicator that there is difference in pathophysiology between RA and OA synovitis. If it is accepted that synovial inflammation, and the production of proinflammatory and destructive mediators from the OA synovium, is of importance for the symptoms and progression of osteoarthritis, it is a key question which cell type in the OA synovium is responsible for maintaining synovial inflammation. In RA, macrophage-produced TNFα is a major therapeutic target, but much less is known about macrophage biology in OA, although histological studies have demonstrated that OA synovial macrophages exhibit an activated phenotype and that they produce both proinflammatory cytokines and vascular endothelial growth factor [46, 50].

The spontaneous production of a variety of pro- and anti-inflammatory cytokines, including TNFα, IL-1β and IL-10, is one of the characteristics of synovial cell cultures derived from digested RA or OA synovium. In addition, the major MMPs and TIMPs are spontaneously produced by these cell cultures [47, 48]. Less TNFα and IL-10 is produced from OA samples, but the levels are still easily detectable by ELISA [48]. It is possible to use effective adenoviral gene transfer in this model without causing apoptosis or disrupting intracellular signalling pathways. Using an adenovirus effectively transferring the inhibitory subunit IκBα, it was possible to selectively inhibit the transcription factor NFκB in synovial cocultures from RA or OA patients. Macrophage-produced TNFα and IL-1β were very strongly NFκB dependent in the RA synovium, but in OA synovium, adenoviral transfer of IκBα did not affect IL-1β production and had only a partial effect on TNFα. Effects on other cytokines were similar in RA and OA synovium, with IL-6 and IL-8 both being NFκB dependent, as well as the p75 soluble TNF receptor, whereas IL-10 and the IL-1 receptor antagonists were both NFκB independent. In addition, the matrix metalloproteinases (MMP) 1, 3 and 13 were strongly NFκB dependent in both RA and OA, but their main inhibitor, tissue inhibitor of metalloproteinases (TIMP)-1, was not [48]. The differential effect of NFκB downregulation on the spontaneous production of TNFα and IL-1β on RA and in OA would indicate that the regulation of at least one key intracellular pathway differs fundamentally between these diseases. It is known that both TNFα and IL-1β have functional NFκB elements on their promoters and that in various macrophage models, there are both NFκB-dependent and NFκB-independent ways of inducing TNFα and IL-1β [51, 52]. It would seem as if there are fundamental differences in the regulation of macrophage-produced TNFα and IL-1β between RA and OA, with cytokine levels being higher and NFκB playing a more important role in RA [48, 51, 53].

In the abovementioned model of cultures of osteoarthritis synovial cells, specific depletion of synovial macrophages could be achieved using incubation of the cells with anti-CD14-conjugated magnetic beads [54]. These CD14+-depleted cultures of synovial cells no longer produced significant amounts of macrophage-derived cytokines like TNFα and IL-1β. Interestingly, there was also significant inhibition (40–70 %) of several cytokines produced mainly by synovial fibroblasts, like IL-6 and IL-8, and also significant downregulation of MMP-1 and MMP-3. This would indicate that OA synovial macrophages play an important role in activating fibroblasts in these densely plated cultures of synovial cells and in perpetuating the production of proinflammatory cytokines and destructive enzymes. That the regulation is not tighter than observed is probably because the fibroblasts have an activated phenotype when put into culture, with considerable spontaneous production of cytokines and other mediators. It can be speculated that once the macrophages are removed, the synovial fibroblasts change their phenotype and downregulate their production of both proinflammatory cytokines and destructive MMPs. To investigate the mechanisms involved in this macrophage-driven stimulation of inflammatory and degradative pathways in the OA synovium, specific neutralisation of the endogenous production of TNFα and/or IL-1β was used in the cultures of OA synovial cell [54]. OA synovial cell cultures were either left untreated, incubated with the p75 TNF soluble receptor Ig fusion protein etanercept (Enbrel), incubated with a neutralising anti-IL-1β antibody or incubated with a combination of Enbrel and anti-IL-1β. As could be expected, TNFα production was effectively neutralised by Enbrel treatment and IL-1β by treatment with the neutralising anti-IL-1β antibody. There was no effect of Enbrel on IL-1β production nor did the neutralising anti-IL-1β antibody affect the production of TNFα. This is in marked contrast to the situation in RA, where IL-1β is strongly TNFα dependent in these cultures of synovial cells [18]. This finding would seem to indicate yet another difference in macrophage cytokine biology between RA and OA: whereas TNFα is the 'boss cytokine' in the RA synovium, regulating the production of IL-1β, there is a redundancy between these two cytokines in the OA synovium, with neither TNFα nor IL-1β regulating the production of the other.

Both Enbrel and the neutralising anti-IL-1β antibody inhibited IL-6 and IL-8, with 60 % inhibition achieved when both IL-1β and TNFα were neutralised. The production of MCP-1 was not affected by the neutralising anti-IL-1β antibody, but it was significantly decreased by Enbrel and by the combination of the two. It was also possible to study the effect of neutralising IL-1β and/or TNFα on the mRNA expression and protein production of the major MMPs and aggrecanases, using RT-PCR and ELISA analysis in parallel [54, 55]. The results indicate that although neither Enbrel nor the neutralising anti-IL-1β antibody had an impressive effect on the important collagenases MMP-1 and MMP-13, combination of the two led to significant inhibition both on the mRNA and protein levels. These findings indicate that in the OA synovium, the macrophages potently regulate the production of several important fibroblast-produced cytokines and MMPs, via a combined effect of IL-1β and TNFα. There was no effect of either Enbrel or the neutralising anti-IL-1β antibody on ADAMTS5 expression, nor was it at all affected by a combination of these treatments. Thus, ADAMTS5 appears to be constitutive in OA synovial cells. In contrast, ADAMTS4 was significantly ($p < 0.05$) inhibited by Enbrel and more potently ($p < 0.01$) inhibited by a combination of Enbrel and the neutralising anti-IL-1β antibody. This would indicate that in the human OA synovium, the upregulation of ADAMTS4 is dependent on TNFα and IL-1 produced by the synovial macrophages, whereas the level of ADAMTS5 is not changed by these cytokines [54, 55]. Thus, there is good evidence that in OA synovium and cartilage, ADAMTS4 is the aggrecanase induced by proinflammatory cytokines, whereas ADAMTS5 appears to be constitutive [54–58]. If it is accepted that OA is a cytokine-driven disease, as indicated by some recent papers suggesting that macrophage-produced IL-1 and TNF play a role in driving destructive responses in OA, this finding would render it likely that ADAMTS4 is the aggrecanase responsible for aggrecanolysis in OA. This is a finding of some importance for the debate regarding the major aggrecanase in OA, which is still ongoing. In murine models of degenerative joint disease, ADAMTS5 is the pathologically induced aggrecanase. Mice lacking ADAMTS4 develop normally and develop surgically induced OA in a similar manner to wild-type mice, but deletion of ADAMTS5 protects mice from developing OA [59–61]. However, there is a discrepancy between human and murine cells with regard to the regulation of ADAMTS4 [62, 63]. If the human, but not murine, ADAMTS4 gene responds to IL-1 stimulation, this brings into question the use of a murine model for the study of human aggrecanolysis, particularly since the normal function of at least ADAMTS5 appears to differ between rodents and primates, the enzyme having vital importance for versican turnover and myofibroblast differentiation in monkeys [64].

An important series of papers using injections of liposome-encapsulated clodronate to induce depletion of synovial lining macrophages has provided some intriguing new information about the role of macrophages in driving degenerative changes in a mouse model of experimental OA induced by injection of collagenase. The collagenase injection causes weakening of ligaments leading to gradual onset of OA pathology within 6 weeks of induction, without any direct collagenase-induced cartilage damage being observed. If macrophage depletion had been achieved prior to the elicitation of experimental OA, there was potent reduction of both fibrosis and osteophyte formation [65, 66]. This would indicate that in this murine model of OA, synovial macrophages control the production of the growth factors that promote fibrosis and osteophyte formation, both key pathophysiological events in OA. In the same mouse model of OA, it was also possible to monitor the effect of macrophage depletion on the formation of the VDIPEN neoepitope that indicates MMP-induced cleavage of aggrecan [49, 67]. Some marginal VDIPEN expression could be observed already on day 7 after induction of collagen-induced arthritis, but there was only a slight decrease in macrophage-depleted joints. Between day 7 and day 14, however, VDIPEN expression more than doubled in non-depleted joints, whereas it remained unchanged in depleted ones. This would indicate that, in agreement with the data from human OA synovium discussed above, the production of MMPs in this murine model of OA is macrophage dependent. Analysis of samples of synovium and cartilage from the murine OA joints in this model demonstrated that MMP-2, 3 and 9 were induced in both these tissues when murine OA was induced by collagenase. But whereas the MMP levels in the cartilage were unaffected by macrophage depletion, those in the synovium were inhibited, suggesting that removal of the macrophages would downregulate the production of MMPs from the synovial fibroblasts and that the gradual decrease in the diffusion of these MMPs to the cartilage would prevent aggrecanolysis, as evidenced by the reduction in VDIPEN expression. In the same model of murine OA, MMP-3 knockout mice showed a 67 % reduction in the occurrence of severe cartilage damage, with a concomitant decrease in VDIPEN expression, indicating involvement of this MMP in the OA disease process [67]. This is a somewhat unexpected and controversial finding, since other studies have indicated an important role for the collagenase MMP-13 in OA. This enzyme is strongly upregulated in the OA synovium [49, 68], and there is a correlation between MMP-13 levels and cartilage damage in human OA, as evidenced by arthroscopy [68]. It may well be that several MMPs contribute to the OA disease process, with an intricate network between proMMPs and their activators.

'After the success of targeted biological therapy in RA, there was a good deal of interest in investigating anti-cytokine strategies also in OA. In a patient with inflammatory knee OA, with synovitis visible on an MRI scan, an anti-TNF biologic had marked benefit on pain and walking distance, as well as synovitis, synovial effusion and bone marrow oedema [69]. In another early pilot study, concerning 12 patients with inflammatory hand OA, the anti-TNF antibody adalimumab had no significant effect, however, although some patients improved [70]. With regard to IL-1, an early study in 13 patients with knee OA has indicated that intra-articular administration of the interleukin-1 receptor antagonist had some degree of analgesic effect [71]. A later double-blind, placebo-controlled study could demonstrate no improvement in knee OA symptoms after intra-articular injection of anakinra, however [72]. Thus, early results from anti-cytokine therapy in OA are not greatly impressive. The immediate effect of anti-TNF biologics in RA, with regard to inflammation, pain and fatigue, has not been reproduced in OA [73]. Although it is likely that a subgroup of patients with knee OA, with bone marrow oedema and synovitis visible on MRI, have benefit from either anti-TNF of anti-IL-1 strategies, the majority of patients, with significant irreversible bone and cartilage damage, the effect of these biologics would be less impressive. As with all potential disease-modifying strategies in OA, a major obstacle for anti-cytokine therapy in OA will be the difficulty of recruiting patients with early inflammatory OA before gross bone and cartilage loss is obvious on X-rays and clinical examination.

The revolution in drug discovery for RA, with not only anti-TNF biologics but also effective anti-B-cell, anti-IL-6 and anti-T cell co-stimulation drugs gaining prominence, has led to more energetic work in the struggle to identify therapeutic targets in OA. None of the older drug candidates, including diacerein, doxycycline, licifelone, risedronate and strontium ranelate, could be clearly demonstrated to have clinical benefit in OA [3, 4], nor have the widely available 'nutraceuticals' glucosamine and chondroitin sulphate been proven to affect either joint pain or joint space narrowing in human OA [5]. The concept that macrophage-produced cytokines from the inflamed synovium play a role in driving inflammatory and destructive pathways in OA was a novel one when first suggested, but much has since been written on this subject, and it appears that the contribution of macrophage-driven synovitis contributing to OA pathogenesis has become widely accepted [7, 8, 74–77]. The problem of making clinical use of this concept has failed, however, with the anti-IL-1 and anti-TNF biologics not being efficacious in established hand or knee OA, particularly in patients without evidence of active synovitis. A number of other potential therapeutic targets in OA have been defined in recent years, one of them the ADAMTS5 metalloproteinase. A study of the monoclonal antibody CRB0017, directed against the spacer domain of ADAMTS5, showed that in a spontaneous murine OA model in STR/ort mice, intra-articular administration of this antibody significantly prevented disease progression in a dose-dependent manner [78]. There was no comparison with systemic administration, nor was it assessed to what degree the antibody leaked from the synovial space. Another study found that systemic administration of the anti-ADAMTS5 antibody GSK2394002 in a model of surgically induced murine OA demonstrated both structural disease modification and alleviation of pain-related behaviour [79]. The effect of GSK2394002 on cardiovascular physiology was carefully monitored in cynomolgus monkeys, and it was found that a single administration of the antibody caused increased mean arterial pressure, and ST elevations on the ECG indicating cardiac ischemia, effects that were sustained for up to 8 months after administration of the single dose [64]. These side effects were considered too formidable to allow for further clinical development of GSK2394002. Another potential therapeutic target was the inducible nitric oxide synthetase (iNOS). In murine joint instability-induced OA, iNOS-deficient mice developed significantly less OA lesions than wild-type mice, with 50 % reduction of both osteophytes and cartilage lesions [80]. In a canine model of

OA induced by joint instability, treatment with the oral selective iNOS inhibitor cindunistat led to significant reduction of OA lesions. Still, a recent clinical study of cindunistat in patients with symptomatic osteoarthritis of the knee showed no significant benefit [81]. Another potential therapeutic target in OA is fibroblast growth factor-18 (sprifermin), which promotes cartilage development and repair. In a rat model of OA, intra-articular injections of sprifermin induced a significant, dose-dependent reduction in cartilage degeneration. In a recent clinical study, sprifermin had no effect on medial femorotibial compartment cartilage volume, although it did significantly and dose dependently reduce the loss of total and lateral femorotibial compartment cartilage volume [82]. In stark contrast to the situation in RA, where there is almost an embarrassment of riches when it comes to both biologics and small-molecule targeted therapy, the search for a disease-modifying anti-osteoarthritis drug has thus far ended in disappointment, with a number of promising drug candidates failing clinical trials.

2.4   Discussion

Radiosynovectomy [also known as 'radiosynoviorthesis' in continental Europe] consists of an intra-articular injection of radionuclides in colloidal form, as local therapy for chronic large-joint synovitis that is refractory to other treatment [83–85]. Both large and small joints can be treated, but in normal clinical practice, the knee and hip predominate. Radiosynovectomy has been used since 1952, and the radionuclide yttrium-90 has been preferred for knee radiosynovectomies since the 1970s, due to strong β radiation and little γ-radiation. It has been difficult to evaluate the technique using double-blind clinical trials, although two trials show superiority of yttrium-90 knee radiosynovectomy over intra-articular triamcinolone [86] or methylprednisolone acetate [87].

Indications for radiosynovectomy include rheumatoid arthritis, other forms of chronic inflammatory arthritis like psoriatic arthritis or ankylosing spondylitis with peripheral joint involvement, haemophilic synovitis and inflammatory osteoarthritis. The procedure has an established niche in hemophilic arthropathy, where surgical synovectomy is not an alternative; it has been proven to reduce the number of bleeding episodes, the joint pain and the degree of clinical synovitis [88]. In spite of the improved treatment of inflammatory arthritis, with a number of effective biologics available, radiosynovectomy also has indications in these diseases, in cases of chronic mono- or oligoarthritis refractory to conventional treatment, including DRARMs, biologics and intra-articular steroids. The use of radiosynovectomy in osteoarthritis is rather more controversial. A New Zealand study showed that while yttrium-90 radiosynovectomy was safe and moderately effective in inflammatory arthritides of the knee, it was of little benefit in established OA, or in patients with secondary OA changes on X-rays [83]. A German study showed good or excellent improvement in clinical symptoms in 40 % of 35 patients with therapy-resistant joint effusions caused by severe OA [89]. A recent Greek study showed a good response to yttrium-90 knee radiosynovectomy in OA patients, with clinical improvement inversely related to radiographic knee damage, patient age and duration of disease [90].

As pointed out earlier in this chapter, the disease mechanisms on RA and in OA are completely different. In RA, there are more synovial macrophages, driving synovial inflammation and development of erosions through TNFα; in OA, there are much fewer synovial macrophages, driving other inflammatory and destructive mediators through TNFα and IL-1, with neither cytokine being the dominant one. Early OA is likely to be quite a different disease to late-stage OA, with severe destruction of cartilage, and involvement of subchondral bone. A radiosynovectomy is likely to be effective in both RA and OA, through depleting synovial macrophages that drive the synovial inflammation through their respective cytokines. There is no reason that a radiosynovectomy should not be effective in early inflammatory OA. As suggested by two clinical studies [83, 90], it is less likely to be effective in 'dry' osteoarthritis with little or no inflammatory component or in patients with irreversible OA damage.

References

1. Kinne RW, Stuhlmuller B, Burmester G-R. Cells of the synovium in rheumatoid arthritis: macrophages. Arthritis Res Ther. 2007;9:224.
2. Feldmann M, Maini RN. Role of cytokines in rheumatoid arthritis: an education in pathophysiology and therapeutics. Immunol Rev. 2008;223:7–19.
3. Hellio Le Graverand-Gastineau M-P. Disease-modifying osteoarthritis drugs: facing development challenges and choosing molecular targets. Curr Drug Targets. 2010;11:528–35.
4. Bondeson J. Are we moving in the right direction with osteoarthritis drug discovery? Expert Opin Ther Targets. 2011;15:1355–68.
5. Wandel S, Juni P, Tendal B, et al. Effects of glucosamine, chondroitin, or placebo in patients with osteoarthritis of hip or knee: network meta-analysis. BMJ. 2010;341:c4675.
6. Bondeson J. Activated synovial macrophages as targets for osteoarthritis drug therapy. Curr Drug Targets. 2010;11:576–85.
7. Scanzello CR, Goldring SR. The role of synovitis in osteoarthritis pathogenesis. Bone. 2012;51:249–57.
8. De Lange-Brokaar BJE, Ioan-Facsinay A, van Osch GJVM, et al. Synovial inflammation, immune cells and their cytokines in osteoarthritis: a review. Osteoarthritis Cartilage. 2012;20:1484–99.
9. Bondeson J, Blom A, Wainwright S, et al. The role of synovial macrophages and macrophage-produced mediators in driving inflammatory and destructive responses in osteoarthritis. Arthritis Rheum. 2010;52:647–57.
10. Sokolove J, Lepus CM. Role of inflammation in the pathogenesis of osteoarthritis: latest findings and interpretations. Ther Adv Musculoskelet Dis. 2013;5:77–94.
11. Bondeson J. The mechanisms of action of disease-modifying antirheumatic drugs: a review with emphasis on macrophage signal transduction and the induction of proinflammatory cytokines. Gen Pharmacol. 1997;29:127–50.
12. Danning CL, Boumpas DT. Commonly used disease-modifying antirheumatic drugs in the treatment of inflammatory arthritis: an update on mechanisms of action. Clin Exp Rheumatol. 1998;16:595–604.
13. Erhardt CC, Mumford PA, Venables PJ, Maini RN. Factors predicting a poor life prognosis in rheumatoid arthritis: an eight year prospective study. Ann Rheum Dis. 1989;48:7–13.
14. Pincus T, Callahan LF. What is the natural history of rheumatoid arthritis? Rheum Dis Clin North Am. 1993;19:123–51.

15. Sack U, Stiehl P, Geiler G. Distribution of macrophages in the rheumatoid synovial membrane and its association with basic activity. Rheumatol Int. 1994;13:181–6.
16. Mulherin D, Fitzgerald O, Bresnihan B. Synovial tissue macrophage populations and articular damage in rheumatoid arthritis. Arthritis Rheum. 1996;39:115–24.
17. Chu CQ, Field M, Allard S, Maini RN. Detection of cytokines at the cartilage/pannus junction in patients with rheumatoid arthritis: implications of the role of cytokines in cartilage destruction and repair. Br J Rheumatol. 1992;31:653–61.
18. Brennan FM, Chantry D, Jackson A, et al. Inhibitory effect of TNFα antibodies on synovial cell interleukin-1 production in rheumatoid arthritis. Lancet. 1989;ii:244–7.
19. Butler DM, Maini RN, Feldmann M, Brennan FM. Modulation of proinflammatory cytokine release in rheumatoid synovial membrane cultures: comparison between monoclonal anti-TNFα antibody with the interleukin-1 receptor antagonist. Eur Cytokine Netw. 1995;6:225–30.
20. Haworth C, Brennan FM, Chantry D, et al. Expression of granulocyte-macrophage colony-stimulating factor (GM-CSF) in rheumatoid arthritis: regulation by tumour necrosis factor α. Eur J Immunol. 1991;21:2575–9.
21. Feldmann M, Brennan FM, Maini RN. Role of cytokines in rheumatoid arthritis. Annu Rev Immunol. 1996;14:397–440.
22. Piguet PF, Grau GE, Vesin C, et al. Evolution of collagen arthritis in mice is arrested by treatment with anti-tumour necrosis factor (TNF) antibody or a recombinant soluble TNF receptor. Immunology. 1992;77:510–4.
23. Williams RO, Feldmann M, Maini RN. Anti-tumour necrosis factor ameliorates joint disease in murine collagen-induced arthritis. Proc Natl Acad Sci U S A. 1992;89:9784–8.
24. Elliott MJ, Mainin RN, Feldmann M, et al. Treatment of rheumatoid arthritis with chimeric antibodies to tumour necrosis factor α. Arthritis Rheum. 1993;36:1681–90.
25. Elliott MJ, Maini RN, Feldmann M, et al. Randomised double-blind comparison of chimeric monoclonal antibody to tumour necrosis factor α. Lancet. 1994;344:1105–10.
26. Maini RN, Breedveld FC, Kalden JR, et al. Therapeutic efficacy of multiple intravenous infusions of anti-tumour necrosis factor α monoclonal antibody combined with low-dose weekly methotrexate in rheumatoid arthritis. Arthritis Rheum. 1998;41:1552–63.
27. Maini RN, St Clair E, Breedveld FC, et al. Infliximab (chimeric anti-tumour necrosis factor α monoclonal antibody) versus placebo in rheumatoid arthritis: a randomised phase III trial. Lancet. 1999;354:1932–9.
28. Lipsky P, van der Heijde D, St Clair EW, et al. Infliximab and methotrexate in the treatment of rheumatoid arthritis. N Engl J Med. 2000;343:1594–602.
29. Moreland LW, Baumgartner SW, Schiff MH, et al. Treatment of rheumatoid arthritis with a recombinant human tumor necrosis factor receptor (p75)-Fc fusion protein. N Engl J Med. 1997;337:141–7.
30. Weinblatt ME, Kremer JM, Bankhurst AD, et al. A trial of etanercept, a recombinant tumor necrosis factor receptor-Fc fusion protein, in patients with rheumatoid arthritis receiving methotrexate. N Engl J Med. 1999;340:253–9.
31. Feldmann M. Translating molecular insights in autoimmunity into effective therapy. Annu Rev Immunol. 2009;27:1–27.
32. Feldmann M, Williams RO, Paleolog E. What have we learnt from targeted anti-TNF therapy? Ann Rheum Dis. 2010;69 Suppl 1:i97–9.
33. Kay J, Fleischmann R, Keystone E, et al. Golimumab 3-year safety update: an analysis of pooled data from the long-term extensions of randomised, double-blind, placebo-controlled trials conducted in patients with rheumatoid arthritis, psoriatic arthritis or ankylosing spondylitis. Ann Rheum Dis. 2015;74:538–46.
34. Gabay C, Emery P, van Vollenhoven R, et al. Tocilizumab monotherapy versus adalimumab monotherapy for treatment of rheumatoid arthritis (ADACTA): a randomised, double-blind, controlled phase 4 trial. Lancet. 2013;381:1541–50.
35. Foxwell B, Browne K, Bondeson J, et al. Efficient adenoviral infection with IkappaB alpha reveals that macrophage tumor necrosis factor alpha production in rheumatoid arthritis is NF-kappaB dependent. Proc Natl Acad Sci U S A. 1998;95:8211–5.

36. Tas SW, Vervoordeldonk MJ, Hajji N, et al. Local treatment with the selective IkappaB kinase beta inhibitor NEMO-binding domain peptide ameliorates synovial inflammation. Arthritis Res Ther. 2006;8:R86.

37. Min S-Y, Yan M, Du Y, et al. Intra-articular nuclear factor-kappaB blockade ameliorates collagen-induced arthritis in mice by eliciting regulatory T cells and macrophages. Clin Exp Immunol. 2013;172:217–27.

38. McCann FE, Palfreeman AC, Andrews M, et al. Apremilast, a novel PDE4 inhibitor, inhibits spontaneous production of tumour necrosis factor α from human rheumatoid synovial cells and ameliorates experimental arthritis. Arthritis Res Ther. 2010;12:R107.

39. Maruotti N, Cantatore FP, Crivellato E, et al. Macrophages in rheumatoid arthritis. Histol Histopathol. 2007;22:581–6.

40. Li J, Hsu H-C, Mountz JB. Managing macrophages in rheumatoid arthritis by reform or removal. Curr Rheumatol Rep. 2012;14:445–54.

41. Davignon J-L, Hayder M, Baron M, et al. Targeting monocytes/macrophages in the treatment of rheumatoid arthritis. Rheumatology. 2013;52:590–8.

42. Van der Heijden JW, Oerlemans R, Dijkmans BAC, et al. Folate receptor β as a potential delivery route for novel folate antagonists to macrophages in the synovial tissue of rheumatoid arthritis patients. Arthritis Rheum. 2009;60:12–21.

43. Nagai T, Kyo A, Hasui K, et al. Efficacy of an immunotoxin to folate receptor beta in the intra-articular treatment of antigen-induced arthritis. Arthritis Res Ther. 2012;14:R106.

44. Clark AG, Jordan JM, Vilim V, Renner JB, Dragomir AD, Luta G, et al. Serum cartilage oligomeric protein reflects osteoarthritis presence and severity. Arthritis Rheum. 1999;42:2356–64.

45. Sowers M, Jannausch M, Stein E, Jamadar D, Hochberg M, Lachance L. C-reactive protein as a biomarker of emergent osteoarthritis. Osteoarthritis Cartilage. 2002;10:595–601.

46. Benito MJ, Veale DJ, FitzGerald O, van den Berg WB, Bresnihan B. Synovial tissue inflammation in early and late osteoarthritis. Ann Rheum Dis. 2005;64:1263–7.

47. Bondeson J, Foxwell BMJ, Brennan FM, Feldmann M. A new approach to defining therapeutic targets: blocking NF-κB inhibits both inflammatory and destructive mechanisms in rheumatoid synovium, but spares anti-inflammatory mediators. Proc Natl Acad Sci U S A. 1999;96:5668–73.

48. Amos N, Lauder S, Evans A, Feldmann M, Bondeson J. Adenoviral gene transfer into osteoarthritis synovial cells using the endogenous inhibitor IκBα reveals that most, but not all, inhibitory and destructive mediators, are NFκB dependent. Rheumatology. 2006;45:1201–9.

49. Blom AB, van den Berg WB. The synovium and its role in osteoarthritis. In: Bronner F, Farach-Carson MC, editors. Bone and osteoarthritis, vol. 4. Berlin: Springer; 2007. p. 65–79.

50. Haywood L, McWilliams DF, Pearson CI, et al. Inflammation and angiogenesis in osteoarthritis. Arthritis Rheum. 2003;48:173–7.

51. Bondeson J, Browne KA, Brennan FM, et al. Selective regulation of cytokine induction by adenoviral gene transfer of IκBα into human macrophages: lipopolysaccharide-induced, but not zymosan-induced, proinflammatory cytokines are inhibited, but IL-10 is NFκB independent. J Immunol. 1999;162:2939–45.

52. Hayes AL, Smith C, Foxwell BM, Brennan FM. CD45-induced tumor necrosis factor alpha production in monocytes is phosphatidylinositol 3-kinase-dependent and nuclear factor kappaB-independent. J Biol Chem. 1999;274:33455–61.

53. Andreakos E, Smith C, Kiriakidis S, et al. Heterogenous requirement of IkappaB kinase 2 for inflammatory cytokine and matrix metalloproteinase production in rheumatoid arthritis: implications for therapy. Arthritis Rheum. 2003;48:1901–12.

54. Bondeson J, Wainwright SD, Lauder S, et al. The role of synovial macrophages and macrophage-produced cytokines in driving aggrecanases, matrix metalloproteinases and other destructive and inflammatory responses in osteoarthritis. Arthritis Res Ther. 2006;8:R187.

55. Bondeson J, Wainwright S, Hughes C, Caterson B. The regulation of ADAMTS4 and ADAMTS5 aggrecanases in osteoarthritis: a review. Clin Exp Rheumatol. 2008;26:139–45.

56. Bau B, Gebhard PM, Haag J, Knorr T, Bartnik E, Aigner T. Relative messenger RNA expression profiling of collagenases and aggrecanases in human articular chondrocytes in vivo and in vitro. Arthritis Rheum. 2002;46:2648–57.
57. Pratta MA, Scherle PA, Yang G, Liu RQ, Newton RC. Induction of aggrecanase-1 (ADAM-TS4) by interleukin-1 occurs through activation of constitutively produced protein. Arthritis Rheum. 2003;48:119–33.
58. Bondeson J, Lauder S, Wainwright SD, Amos N, Evans A, Hughes C, et al. Adenoviral gene transfer of the endogenous inhibitor IkappaBalpha into human osteoarthritis synovial fibroblasts demonstrates that several matrix metalloproteinases and aggrecanases are NFkappaB dependent. J Rheumatol. 2007;34:523–33.
59. Glasson SS, Askew R, Sheppard B, et al. Characterization of and osteoarthritis susceptibility in ADAMTS-4-knockout mice. Arthritis Rheum. 2004;50:2547–58.
60. Glasson SS, Askew R, Sheppard B, et al. Deletion of active ADAMTS5 prevents cartilage degradation in a murine model of osteoarthritis. Nature. 2005;434:644–8.
61. Stanton H, Rogerson FM, East CJ, et al. ADAMTS5 is the major aggrecanase in mouse cartilage in vivo and in vitro. Nature. 2005;434:648–52.
62. East CJ, Stanton H, Golub SB, et al. ADAMTS-5 deficiency does not block aggrecanolysis at preferred cleavage sites in the chondroitin sulfate rich region of aggrecan. J Biol Chem. 2007;282:8632–40.
63. Zwerina J, Redlich K, Polzer K, et al. TNF-induced structural joint damage is mediated by IL-1. Proc Natl Acad Sci U S A. 2007;104:11742–7.
64. Larkin J, Lohr T, Elefante L, et al. The highs and lows of translational drug development: antibody-mediated inhibition of ADAMTS-5 for osteoarthritis disease modification. Osteoarthritis Cartilage. 2014;22iii:S483.
65. Blom AB, van Lent PLEM, Holthuysen AEM, van der Kraan PM, Roth J, van Rooijen N, et al. Synovial lining macrophages mediate osteophyte formation during experimental osteoarthritis. Osteoarthritis Cartilage. 2004;12:627–35.
66. Van Lent PLEM, Blom AB, van der Kraan P, Holthuysen AEM, Vitters E, van Rooijen N, et al. Crucial role of synovial lining macrophages in the promotion of transforming growth factor beta-mediated osteophyte formation. Arthritis Rheum. 2004;50:103–11.
67. Blom AB, van Lent PL, Libregts S, Holthuysen AE, van der Kraan PM, van Rooijen N, et al. Crucial role of macrophages in matrix metalloproteinase-mediated cartilage destruction during experimental osteoarthritis. Arthritis Rheum. 2007;56:147–57.
68. Marini S, Fasciglione GF, Monteleone G, Maiotti M, Tarantino U, Coletta G. A correlation between knee cartilage degradation observed by arthroscopy and synovial proteinases activity. Clin Biochem. 2003;36:295–304.
69. Grunke M, Schulze-Koops H. Successful treatment of inflammatory knee osteoarthritis with tumour necrosis factor blockade. Ann Rheum Dis. 2006;65:555–6.
70. Magnano MD, Chakravarty EF, Broudy C, Chung L, Kelman A, Hillygus J, et al. A pilot study of tumor necrosis factor inhibition in erosive/inflammatory osteoarthritis of the hands. J Rheumatol. 2007;34:1323–7.
71. Chevalier X, Girardeau B, Conzorier T, Marliere J, Kiefer P, Goupille P. Safety study of intraarticular injection of interleukin 1 receptor antagonist in patients with painful knee osteoarthritis: a multicenter study. J Rheumatol. 2005;32:1317–23.
72. Chevalier X, Goupille P, Beaulieu AD, Burch FX, Bensen WG, Conrozier T, et al. Intraarticular injection of anakinra in osteoarthritis of the knee: a multicenter, double-blind, placebo-controlled study. Arthritis Care Res. 2009;61:344–52.
73. Chevalier X, Eymard F, Richette P. Biologic agents in osteoarthritis: hopes and disappointments. Nat Rev Rheumatol. 2013;9:400–10.
74. Attur M, Samuels J, Krasnokutsky S, Abramson SB. Targeting the synovial tissue for treating osteoarthritis: where is the evidence? Best Pract Res Clin Rheumatol. 2010;24:71–9.
75. Kapoor M, Martel-Pelletier J, Lajeunesse D, et al. Role of proinflammatory cytokines in the pathophysiology of osteoarthritis. Nat Rev Rheumatol. 2011;7:33–42.

76. Martel-Pelletier J, Wildi LM, Pelletier J-P. Future therapeutics for osteoarthritis. Bone. 2012;51:297–311.
77. Haseeb A, Haqqi TM. Immunopathogenesis of osteoarthritis. Clin Immunol. 2013;146:185–96.
78. Chiusaroli R, Visentini M, Galimberti C, et al. Targeting of ADAMTS5's ancillary domain with the recombinant antibody CRB0017 ameliorates disease progression in a spontaneous murine model of osteoarthritis. Osteoarthritis Cartilage. 2013;21:1807–10.
79. Miller RE, Tran PB, Ishihara S, et al. Therapeutic efficacy of anti-ADAMTS5 antibody in the DMM model. Osteoarthritis Cartilage. 2014;22iii:S35.
80. van den Berg WB, van de Loo F, Joosten LA, Arntz OJ. Animal models of arthritis in iNOS-deficient mice. Osteoarthritis Cartilage. 1999;7:413–5.
81. Hellio le Graverand M-P, Clemmer RS, Redifer P, et al. A two-year randomized double-blind, placebo-controlled, multicentre study of oral selective iNOS inhibitor cindunistat (SD-6010) in patients with symptomatic osteoarthritis of the knee. Ann Rheum Dis. 2013;72:187–95.
82. Lohmander LS, Hellot S, Dreher D. Intraarticular sprifermin (recombinant human fibroblast growth factor 18) in knee osteoarthritis: a randomized, double-blind, placebo-controlled trial. Arthritis Rheum. 2014;66:1820–31.
83. Taylor WJ, Corkill MM, Rajapakse CAN. A retrospective review of yttrium-90 synovectomy in the treatment of knee arthritis. Br J Rheumatol. 1997;36:1100–5.
84. Schneider P, Farahati J, Reiners C. Radiosynovectomy in rheumatology, orthopaedics and haemophilia. J Nucl Med. 2005;46 Suppl 1:48S–54.
85. Zwolak R, Majdan M, Skorski M, Chrapko B. Efficacy of radiosynoviorthesis and its impact on chosen inflammatory markers. Rheumatol Int. 2012;32:2339–44.
86. Menkes C, Le Go A, Verrier P, Delbarre F. A controlled trial of intra-articular yttrium-90, osmic acid and triamcinolone hexacetonide in rheumatoid arthritis. XIV Int Congr Rheum San Francisco 1977:614.
87. Szanto E. Long term follow up of yttrium-90 treated knee joints. Scand J Rheumatol. 1978;6:209–12.
88. Rodriguez-Merchan EC, De la Corte-Rodriguez H, Jimenez-Yuste V. Radiosynovectomy in haemophilia: long-term results of 500 procedures performed in a 38-year period. Thromb Res. 2014;134:985–90.
89. Kroger S, Sawula JA, Klutmann S, et al. Efficacy of radiation synovectomy in degenerative inflammatory and chronic inflammatory joint diseases. Nuklearmedizin. 1999;38:279–84.
90. Markou P, Chatzopoulos D. Yttrium-90 silicate radiosynovectomy treatment of painful synovitis in knee osteoarthritis. Hell J Nucl Med. 2009;12:33–6.

Intra-articular Corticosteroid Treatment of Inflammatory Joint Diseases

3

Christopher L. Tracy and Jess D. Edison

Contents

C.L. Tracy • J.D. Edison (✉)
Walter Reed National Military Medical Center, 8901 Rockville Pike, Bethesda, MD 20889, USA
e-mail: Jess.d.edison.mil@health.mil

© Springer International Publishing Switzerland 2015

49

W.U. Kampen, M. Fischer (eds.), *Local Treatment of Inflammatory Joint Diseases: Benefits and Risks*, DOI 10.1007/978-3-319-16949-1_3

3.1   Introduction/History

On January 27, 1951, a study group led by Joseph Lee Hollander injected three rheumatoid arthritis patients with the first intra-articular hydrocortisone injections. These three patients showed clinical improvements in local inflammation. This group went on to inject 1,500 test patients with nearly 24,000 injections into the joints, bursae, and tendon sheaths. Fifty percent of these patients experienced clinically significant improvement of local inflammation [1]. Over the last 65 years, corticosteroid injections have become a valuable and efficacious treatment option in the management of inflammatory arthritis with an excellent safety record [2].

This chapter will provide an overview of the indications for use of corticosteroid injections, the specific agents used, the adverse effects of corticosteroid joint injections, corticosteroid effects on the synovium, and overall efficacy in select types of inflammatory arthropathies.

3.1.1   Indication

The most common indication for intra-articular injections in inflammatory joint disease is the presence of joint pain. Corticosteroids have been used successfully in a number of inflammatory arthritis conditions to include rheumatoid arthritis, crystalline arthropathies (gout and pseudogout), spondyloarthropathies (psoriatic arthritis, ankylosing spondylitis, reactive arthritis, inflammatory bowel disease-associated arthritis), other connective tissue disease-associated arthritis (systemic lupus erythematosus, mixed connective tissue disease, Sjogren's syndrome), and juvenile idiopathic arthritis. Although frequently used in clinical practice, there is little systematic evidence to guide corticosteroid selection for therapeutic injections.

3.1.2   Commonly Used Corticosteroids

Common corticosteroid preparations include topical, oral, and parenteral formulations. Only depot preparations are suitable for joint injections. Depot formulations remain at the injected site for a longer period of time and display mainly localized efficacy. Knowledge of the difference in potency and solubility of injectable corticosteroids is useful for clinical practice since the duration of action of the particular agent is inversely related to the solubility of the preparation – more soluble compounds are thought to have a shorter duration of action [3–5].

3.1.3   Solubility

Solubility is a key factor in efficacy because compounds with lower solubility maintain effective intra-articular therapeutic response longer and produce lower systemic levels of corticosteroid than would compounds of greater solubility. A lower systemic level of corticosteroid is generally viewed as a favorable feature of intra-articular injections because of the potential to reduce systemic toxicity. To support this concept, in a comparison of two preparations with different solubilities, triamcinolone acetonide and triamcinolone hexacetonide, absorption rate was markedly different with the less soluble compound, triamcinolone hexacetonide, and resulted in lower corticosteroid peak plasma levels [6].

3.1.4   Duration of Action

Few controlled long-term studies assess pain relief after intra-articular corticosteroid injections in inflammatory arthritis, and the reported ranges of duration of action vary widely between corticosteroids. Data suggests that decreased solubility correlates with increased duration of action with many depot preparations. In one clinical trial, however, triamcinolone hexacetonide showed less of a clinical effect when injected into osteoarthritic knees than a more soluble compound, methylprednisolone acetate, suggesting that there may be a more complex explanation for duration of action in some disease states [3]. The most durable effect is achieved in the knee of patients with pauciarticular JIA with a mean duration of remission of 13.9 months. This is in contrast to osteoarthritis where the duration of symptom relief is only 3 weeks and function is not improved [4]. Overall, the duration of response has been found to vary according to the type of corticosteroid preparation used, dose, subtype of arthritis, duration of disease prior to the injection, specific joint injected, and accuracy of the injection [4, 7].

3.1.5   Frequency of Injections

Theoretical risks of cartilage loss and subsequent joint replacement are often cited when considering injection frequency. The optimal frequency remains controversial. Raynauld and colleagues showed relative safety with corticosteroid injections every 3 months in a patient population with osteoarthritis [8]. Patients with rheumatoid arthritis receiving up to ten injections in a year on a single joint failed to show significant increase in cartilage loss or need for joint replacement [8, 9]. In clinical practice, the inherent risk of cartilage loss and subsequent need for joint replacement in patients with active inflammation are well understood and often dictate frequency of injection.

3.1.6   Local Anesthetics

Local anesthetics to include lidocaine 1 % and bupivacaine 0.25–0.5 % are commonly mixed with the corticosteroid depot preparation to provide temporary analgesia and dilute the crystalline suspension for improved diffusion within the injection site. Local anesthesia can also be used to diagnostically confirm the correct placement of the preparation by improving pain in the local area with its quick onset of action. Manufactures advise against mixing corticosteroid preparations with lidocaine because of the risk of clumping and precipitation of steroid crystals; however, in clinical practice, lidocaine is a useful diluent. Patients rarely experience side effects directly related to the anesthetic. These side effects occur within 30 min of the injection and include flushing, hives, and chest or abdominal discomfort [5].

3.1.7 Corticosteroid Preparations

The major depot preparations include methylprednisolone acetate, triamcinolone hexacetonide, triamcinolone acetonide, betamethasone acetate/betamethasone sodium phosphate, and betamethasone dipropionate/betamethasone sodium phosphate. All dissolve slower than earlier depot preparations such as hydrocortisone acetate in order to achieve a prolonged local effect [4].

Potency of corticosteroids is measured against that of hydrocortisone and ranges from low-potency short-acting agents to high-potency, long-acting agents.

Hydrocortisone acetate (hydrocortisone acetate, 25 mg/ml) has the shortest duration of action of steroids mentioned in this chapter and is dosed at 10–25 mg for small-joint injections and 50 mg for large-joint injections. It is very soluble and has limited utility in joint injections given its low potency and short duration of action [8].

Methylprednisolone acetate (methylprednisolone acetate 40 mg/ml – concentrated) has intermediate potency and duration of action. It is dosed at 2–10 mg for small-joint injections and 10–80 mg for large-joint injections [8, 9].

Triamcinolone acetonide (triamcinolone acetonide 40 mg/ml – concentrated) has intermediate potency and duration of action and is very similar to methylprednisolone in structure and activity and is dosed similar to methylprednisolone for small- and large-joint injections [8, 9].

Betamethasone sodium phosphate and acetate (betamethasone sodium phosphate and acetate 6 mg/ml) has high potency. This formulation combines a soluble ester (sodium phosphate) to provide prompt activity with a much less soluble betamethasone acetate to obtain sustained duration of activity. It is dosed at 2–6 mg for large joints and 1–3 mg for small joints [8, 9] (Table 3.1).

Table 3.1 Corticosteroid agents by relative potencies [8, 9]

Steroid	Potency	Solubility	Relative anti-inflammatory potency
Hydrocortisone acetate	Low	Soluble	1
Methylprednisolone acetate	Intermediate	Soluble	5
Triamcinolone acetonide	Intermediate	Relatively insoluble	5
Betamethasone sodium phosphate and acetate	High	Combination	25

Table 3.2 Adverse effects following intra-articular corticosteroid injections [3, 4, 20]

Adverse effect	Estimated rate/frequency
Infection	Rare 1:1,000–1:50,000
Capsular calcification	Common 25–50 %
Cutaneous atrophy	Uncommon <1 %
Flushing	Relatively common 1–15 %
Post-injection flare	Relatively common 1–10 %
Tendon rupture	Uncommon <1 %
Osteonecrosis	Uncommon, reported cases

3.1.8 Adverse Events

Although animal studies have suggested that corticosteroid injections may have damaging effects on articular cartilage, human studies have not shown similar results [11, 12]. Intra-articular corticosteroid injections have an excellent safety record, and its safe use is supported by a large body of clinical data. The American College of Rheumatology has endorsed corticosteroid injections as safe and effective when administered by experienced physicians [2]. Despite their relative safe use, known side effects exist. Table 3.2 lists common and uncommon local adverse effects of intra-articular corticosteroids.

The most common reported side effects following corticosteroid injections are post-injection flair, facial flushing, and cutaneous atrophy [13].

3.1.9 Post-injection Flare

Pain in the injected joint or at the site of injection can occur within the first 24 h after injection in up to 10 % of patients. Localized tissue damage resulting from needle puncture may be a partial cause for injection site reactions. More often, though, it is the crystalline structure of the particular corticosteroid agent used that results in a localized synovitis [14].

3.1.10 Facial Flushing

Facial flushing occurs within a few hours post injection in up to 15 % of patients and is particularly common in women. Although benign, symptoms may linger for up to 3–4 days [15].

3.1.11 Cutaneous Atrophy

Skin or fat atrophy following corticosteroid injections usually develops within 1–4 months. It occurs more commonly in patient with juvenile idiopathic arthritis and is reported in up to 8 % of injections [16]. Overall it is thought to occur at a rate of less than 1 % and may be accompanied with depigmentation of the skin [13]. The atrophy and depigmentation is due to the leakage of the injected steroids into the skin and may improve over a few months. It is more likely to occur following the small-joint injections where the accuracy of injection is not guaranteed, the subcutaneous tissue is thinner, and a larger volume of corticosteroids are injected. Less soluble agents are also more likely to cause these cutaneous adverse effects [3, 4].

3.1.12 Capsular Calcification

Capsular calcification is the most common local adverse reaction following an intra-articular corticosteroid injection and occurs in up to 25–50 % of patients but is rarely clinically significant [17]. Pericapsular or intracapsular calcifications are noted within 2 months to 1 year following the injection and are usually asymptomatic. The location of the calcification is related to the site of the needle injection and is composed of hydroxyapatite [4].

3.1.13 Tendon Ruptures

Ruptured tendons occur uncommonly and have been reported in patients following intra-articular corticosteroid injections that have been placed directly within a tendon and may occur following a single injection in nearly 25 % of reported cases. Achilles tendon ruptures make up 50 % of reported cases followed by patellar tendon and biceps tendon ruptures in 19 and 8 % of cases respectively [18]. Great care should be used to avoid inadvertent injections within tendons.

3.1.14 Infections

The risk of causing a joint infection is one of the greatest concerns with the use of intra-articular corticosteroid injections, but it is one of the least common reported side effects. Pal B and Morris J reported the perceived risks of joint infection following intra-articular corticosteroid injections between 1 in 1,000 and 1 in 25,000 among rheumatologists surveyed [19]. The reported incidences in another study following knee injections ranged from 1 in 3,000 to 1 in 50,000 [20].

Systemic side effects on intra-articular injections are generally milder than with oral or intravenous formulations and often of unclear significance when present. Reported systemic side effects of systemic glucocorticoids include weight gain and fat redistribution, osteoporosis and fracture, osteonecrosis, ocular complications, hyperglycemia and diabetes, cardiovascular effects, infection, gastrointestinal complications, steroid-induced myopathy, hypothalamic-pituitary-adrenal axis suppression, and psychiatric complications. Table 3.3 lists drug-referenced side effects of glucocorticoids

Table 3.3 Adverse reactions of glucocorticoids for systemic therapy reported from manufacturers prescribing information

	Adverse reactions
CNS	Euphoria, insomnia, psychotic behavior, pseudotumor cerebri, vertigo, headache, paresthesia, seizures
Cardiovascular	Heart failure, hypertension, edema, arrhythmias, thromboembolism
EENT	Cataracts, glaucoma
GI	Peptic ulceration, GI irritation, increased appetite, pancreatitis, nausea, vomiting
GU	Menstrual irregularities
Hepatic	Liver dysfunction
Metabolic	Hypokalemia, hyperglycemia, carbohydrate intolerance, hypocalcemia
Musculoskeletal	Muscle weakness, osteoporosis
Skin	Delayed wound healing, acne, various skin eruptions, hirsutism
Other	Cushingoid state, immunocompromise, growth suppression in children, acute adrenal insufficiency

3.1.15 Hypothalamic-Pituitary-Adrenal Axis Suppression

Suppression of the hypothalamic-pituitary-adrenal axis following intra-articular injections is well-documented and usually mild and transient [3]. An average of 21.5 % reduction in serum cortisol levels returning to baseline after 72 h has been reported. Less commonly, prolonged HPA axis suppression lasting 5–7 weeks has also been reported [21].

3.1.16 Glucose Intolerance

Increased hepatic glucose synthesis and decreased insulin sensitivity have been shown to occur following corticosteroid therapy [22]. Intra-articular corticosteroid injections cause a transient increase in blood glucose levels; however no changes in fasting or predinner blood glucose readings were identified over a 2-week time period in a report of diabetic patients who received a methylprednisolone acetate injection for rheumatic complaints [23].

3.1.17 Steroid-Induced Myopathy

Steroid-induced myopathy is a known consequence of corticosteroid therapy and is more common with fluorinated corticosteroids (triamcinolone, dexamethasone) than with the non-fluorinated corticosteroids (hydrocortisone and methylprednisolone). It has not been reported following intra-articular injections [24].

3.1.18 Osteonecrosis

Osteonecrosis occurs in 5–40 % of patients treated with oral glucocorticoids with increased incidence at higher doses and longer duration. It is reported rarely in oral doses less than 20 mg/day and has been reported following multiple joint injections within days to months.

3.1.19 Osteoporosis

Osteoporosis is a known side effect of systemic glucocorticoid use. Observational studies report the development of fracture-related bone loss in as high as 40 % of patients with systemic glucocorticoid use [25]. In contrast, no net effect on bone resorption and only a transient effect on bone formation were found in a study following single intra-articular triamcinolone acetonide injections [26]. A theoretic benefit of increased mobility following intra-articular injections may also counteract osteoporotic effects.

3.2　Effects of CSI on Synovium

The rationale for using corticosteroids in the treatment of arthritis is to suppress inflammation, suppress inflammatory flares, and disrupt the inflammatory damage-repair-damage cycle. While the clinical efficacy of intra-articular glucocorticoids is well described, there is very limited data on the effects on human synovial tissue in inflammatory arthritis. The systemic effects of glucocorticoids are well described and mediated by receptor antagonism of nuclear factor kappa beta (NF-kB). NF-kB antagonism results in decreased transcription of several genes involved in the immune inflammatory response. It has also been shown to destabilize mRNA. These effects result in a dramatic reduction in cytokine production yielding pleotropic results to include effects on endothelial cells, cell migration, monocytes, macrophages, neutrophils, eosinophils, lymphocytes, fibroblasts, bone, cartilage, muscle, and the synovial tissue [27]. An in vivo study examining the synovial biopsy tissue of 31 patients with inflammatory arthritis, mostly RA, sheds some light on what happens in the synovium. Synovial protein expression of tumor necrosis factor (TNF), interleukin (IL)-1 beta, extranuclear high-mobility group box protein (HMGB)-1, vascular endothelial growth factor (VEGF), and ICAM-1 was reduced but without significant effects on vascularity [28]. Notably, macrophage infiltration and proinflammatory endothelial cytokine expression were not reduced, possibly explaining the transient nature of improvements with intra-articular corticosteroids. In this study, all patients demonstrated clinical improvements, although it should be noted that many patients were on other DMARDs or systemic corticosteroids [28]. More recently, synovial citrullinated protein has been correlated with the degree of local inflammation. Treatment with intra-articular corticosteroids has been shown to alter the expression of the synovial citrullinated proteins in the inflamed joint.

This downregulation has been correlated with glucocorticoid effects on a specific protein, peptidylarginine deiminase 4 (PAD4). PAD4 activation, induction, and signaling pathway is dependent on NF-kB suggesting glucocorticoids may affect citrullination through PAD4 downregulation in an NF-kB-dependent pathway [29, 30]. A summary of the described cellular effects following glucocorticoids is listed in Table 3.4.

Table 3.4 Cellular effects following glucocorticoid administration [27]

Endothelial cells and cell migration	Inhibits MHC class II antigen, ICAM-1, ELAM-1, E-selectin, TNF-α, IL-1, IL-6, and COX-2 expression; inhibits nitric oxide, arachidonic acid metabolites, complement proteins, and angiogenesis. Blocks endothelin receptor expression, stabilizes vascular permeability, upregulates lipocortin 1
Monocytes, macrophages, and neutrophils	Inhibit neutrophil functions of superoxide generation, chemotaxis, adhesion, apoptosis, and phagocytosis; inhibit arachidonic acid metabolites
	Decrease migration to sites of inflammation
	Induce lipocortin 1, lipomodulin, macrocortin
	Inhibit macrophage antigen presentation to T lymphocytes
	Suppress NF-kB and COX-2
	Inhibit production of cytokines (e.g. IL-1, TNF, IL-6)
	Decrease monocyte Fc receptors
	Decrease Fc receptors on phagocytes
Eosinophils	Decrease migration to sites of inflammation
Lymphocytes	Induce lymphopenia due to redistribution (e.g., in the bone marrow) of lymphoctyes
	Decrease IL-2 and IFNγ production and signal transduction
	Regulate thymopoiesis, primarily via apoptosis
	Inhibit T cell function and natural killer cell activity
	Suppress T cell function and natural killer cell activity
Fibroblast	Decrease proliferation and protein synthesis
	Decrease synthesis and metalloproteinases (e.g., stromelysin and collagenase)
	Inhibit IL-6, IL-8, and GM-CSF
Bone	Inhibit bone formation, inhibit osteoblast function, increase osteoclast life span and function
Cartilage (chondrocytes)	Increase glycosaminoglycan and DNA synthesis
Muscle	Induce atrophy
Synovium	Decrease expression of collagenase, TIMP, PIIINP, TNF, IL-8, E-selectin, ICAM-1, hyaluronate, CCP

MHC major histocompatibility complex, *ICAM-1* intercellular adhesion molecule 1, *ELAM-1* endothelial leukocyte adhesion molecule 1, *TNF* tumor necrosis factor, *IL-1* interleukin-1, *COX-2* cyclooxygenase 2, *NF-kB* nuclear factor kB, *IFNγ* interferon-γ. *GM-CSF* granulocyte-macrophage colony-stimulating factor, *TIMP* tissue inhibitor of metalloproteinase, *PIIINP* N-propeptide of type III procollagen

3.3   Efficacy

3.3.1   Rheumatoid Arthritis

Clinical results following intra-articular corticosteroid injections show immediate effect and demonstrate decreased synovial membrane volume within the first 24 h. Mean duration of improvement is up to 8-week duration following knee joint injection. Reduction in PMN leukocyte number and decrease in pannus size have been shown [4]. Following knee joint corticosteroid injections, patients show significant improvement in pain, morning stiffness of the injected knee, and decreased circumference of the knee and improved range of motion and walking distance when assessed at 1 and 3 months with no benefit with rest following injection [31].

The failure of IAGC to modulate disease, however, has also been noted in a small study evaluating the effects of IAGC with MRI and US. Intra-articular glucocorticoid injection into the wrist failed to arrest bone marrow edema or progression of erosions in rheumatoid arthritis when assessed by MRI and ultrasound at 4 weeks post injection; however, the patients enjoyed a significant clinical response [32].

3.3.2   Juvenile Idiopathic Arthritis (JIA)

Juvenile idiopathic arthritis is a heterogeneous group of disorders, and the use of intra-articular corticosteroids for treatment of joint inflammation can provide significant relief of pain and improved overall function in regard to walking velocity, joint movement, and gait pattern [33]. Patients who receive intra-articular corticosteroids as the primary therapy for oligoarticular JIA were less likely to experience localized growth disturbances versus NSAIDs alone [34]. Total remission has been shown in greater than 80 % of patients with a mean duration of nearly 15 months in patients with knee involvement [35]. Sustained remission has been found in patients with higher ESR and earlier treatment interventions. Shorter duration of efficacy has been found in patients with higher synovial fluid PMN% and + ANA status [36]. Unlike adult rheumatoid arthritis, there is evidence to support knee rest following intra-articular corticosteroid injections. MRI has shown long-lasting suppression of inflammation and pannus without evidence of cartilage destruction. Concern exists regarding the impact on growth in children exposed to corticosteroids, but there is currently no evidence to support any effect on statural growth with IAGC injections [37].

Multiple published reports have shown increased duration of efficacy with the use of less soluble corticosteroid preparations. The less soluble triamcinolone hexacetonide (THA) has shown to have superior efficacy to more soluble depot preparations, betamethasone and triamcinolone acetonide; however, increased rates of cutaneous/subcutaneous atrophy occurred with the less soluble depot formulation, THA, and ranged from 2.3 to 8.3 % [34, 38].

3.3.3 Spondyloarthropathy

Inflammatory back pain and sacroiliitis are major clinical features of a heterogeneous group of inflammatory disorders: seronegative spondyloarthropathy. Conventional treatments which include nonsteroidal anti-inflammatory drugs (NSAIDs) and disease-modifying antirheumatic drugs (DMARDs) are not completely effective. NSAIDs and physiotherapy have been shown to be only partially effective as noted in a 1992 analysis in patients with ankylosing spondylitis [39]. In more recent studies, antitumor necrosis factor-α (TNF-α) agents have shown significant and sustained improvements in symptoms [40]. Many studies have shown efficacy with the use of intra-articular glucocorticoid treatments into the sacroiliac joint in the treatment of spondyloarthropathies. In one published review of 30 patients receiving CT-guided IACI at the sacroiliac joint using 40 mg of triamcinolone acetonide, 83 % had a significant reduction in back pain symptoms lasting greater than 8 months. Magnetic resonance imaging was completed to evaluate for inflammation and showed a mean duration of significant improvement of inflammation lasting 5.2 months [41]. In a meta-analysis, 58–90 % of patients showed greater than 6-month improvement of sacroiliitis following intra-articular corticosteroid injections [4]. Prevention of disease-related joint damage regardless of mode of therapy remains to be shown [42].

3.3.4 Crystalline Arthropathy

Crystalline arthropathies to include gout and pseudogout are inflammatory disorders characterized by the deposition of crystals in synovial fluid and other tissues resulting in exquisitely painful, inflammatory arthritis affecting one or more joints. Although the safety and efficacy of glucocorticoids has been established in other inflammatory arthropathies, there is little or no published evidence to support their safety and efficacy in this setting as noted in a 2013 systematic review [43]. Despite this lack of published evidence to establish efficacy, the use of intra-articular corticosteroid injections for acute gout remains an established therapeutic intervention and is deemed highly effective [44] (Table 3.5).

Table 3.5 Clinical efficacy following intra-articular injections [4, 44, 49]

Rheumatoid arthritis	
Knee	Improved pain and ROM for 1–3 months
Wrist	Improved tender joint score for 4 weeks
Juvenile idiopathic arthritis	
Knee	Remission in pauciarticular for >6 months
Seronegative spondyloarthritis	
Sacroiliac	Subjective improvements lasting up to 10 months
Crystalline arthritis (gout)	
Knee	Resolution of symptoms at 48 h with single injection

3.3.5 Musculoskeletal Ultrasound

Using physical exam techniques by palpating the surface anatomy, skilled orthopedic surgeons and rheumatologist have shown poor accuracy on proper needle placement for intra-articular corticosteroid treatments. Unintended non-intra-articular injection rates are as high as 50–60 % [45–47]. In contrast, sonographic image guidance has shown to improve accuracy with proper positioning of the needle in up to 96–100 % accuracy [47, 48]. Integration of image-guided procedures into clinical practice, however, has been slowed due to the limited evidence supporting improved outcomes using sonography relative to palpation techniques. In a more recently published review, 148 patients were randomized to IA triamcinolone acetonide injection by conventional palpation – versus sonographic image – guided technique. Relative to conventional palpation technique, sonographic needle guidance resulted in 43 % reduction in procedural pain, 58.5 % reduction in absolute pain scores at 2-week follow-up, 25 % increase in the responder rate, and 62 % decrease in the nonresponder rate. Sonography also increased the detection of effusion by 200 % and resulted in the increased volume of aspirated fluid by 337 % [47].

Conclusion

Intra-articular glucocorticoid injections have been used enthusiastically and successfully since 1951, but much remains to be understood regarding their optimal use in clinical practice. A large body of clinical trial data supports the efficacy of intra-articular corticosteroid injections. Used appropriately, injectable corticosteroids can improve pain and allow patients to regain mobility, but wide variability exists in their efficacy in any given disease state. IAGCs are generally safe with rare occurrences of serious adverse events such as infection or avascular necrosis. Despite their long history of use, questions remain concerning the comparative effectiveness and safety of different preparations in various conditions. Factors affecting the durability of treatment effects are also incompletely understood, and a better understanding may lead to more effective therapeutic agents in the future [3].

References

1. Hollander JL. The use of intra-articular hydrocortisone, its analogs, and its higher esters in arthritis. Ann N Y Acad Sci. 1955;61:511–6.
2. Guidelines, American College of Rheumatology Subcommittee on Rheumatoid Arthritis. Guidelines for the management of rheumatoid arthritis: 2002 update. Arthritis Rheum. 2002;46:328–46.
3. Cole BJ, Schumacher Jr HR. Injectable corticosteroids in modern practice. J Am Acad Orthop Surg. 2005;13:37–46.
4. Habib GS, Saliba W, Nashashibi M. Local effects of intra-articular corticosteroids. Clin Rheumatol. 2010;29:347–56.
5. Cordone DA, Tallia E. Joint and soft tissue injection. Am Fam Physician. 2002;66:283–8.
6. Derendorf H, et al. Pharmacokinetics and pharmacodynamics of glucocorticoid suspensions after intra-articular administration. Clin Pharmacol Ther. 1986;39:313–7.

7. Dent PB, Walker N. Intra-articular corticosteroids in the treatment of juvenile rheumatoid arthritis. Curr Opin Rheumatol. 1998;10:475–80.
8. Saunders S, Longworth S. Injection techniques in musculoskeletal medicine. Edinburg: Churchill Livingstone; 2012.
9. Schumacher HR, Chen LX. Injectable corticosteroids in treatment of arthritis of the knee. Am J Med. 2005;118:1208–14.
10. Stephens M, Beutler A, O'Connor F. Musculoskeletal injections: a review of the evidence. Am Fam Physician. 2008;78:971–5.
11. Raynauld JP, Buckland-Wright C, Ward E, et al. Safety and efficacy of long-term intraarticular steroid injections in osteoarthritis of the knee: a randomized, double blind, placebo-controlled trial. Arthritis Rheum. 2003;48:370–7.
12. Roberts WN, Babcock EA, Breitbach SA, et al. Corticosteroid injection in rheumatoid arthritis does not increase rate of total joint arthroplasty. J Rheumatol. 1996;23:1001–4.
13. Kumar N, Newman RJ. Complications of intra- and peri-articular steroid injections. Br J Gen Pract. 1999;49:465–6.
14. Kahn CB, Hollander JL, Schumacher HR. Corticosteroid crystals in synovial fluid. JAMA. 1970;211:807–9.
15. Firetein GS, Panayi GS, Wollheim FA. Rheumatoid arthritis frontiers in pathogenesis and treatment. Oxford: Oxford University Press; 2000. p. 361–9.
16. Cassidy JT, Bole GG. Cutaneous atrophy secondary to intra-articular glucocorticoid administration. Ann Intern Med. 1966;65:1008–18.
17. Gilsanz V, Bernstein BH. Joint calcification following intra-articular corticosteroid therapy. Radiology. 1984;151:647–9.
18. Blanco I, Krahenbuhl S, Schlienger RG. Corticosteroid-associated tendinopathies: an analysis of the published literature and spontaneous pharmacovigilance data. Drug Saf. 2005;28:633–43.
19. Pal B, Morris J. The perceived risks of joint injection following intra-articular corticosteroid injections: a survey of rheumatologists. Clin Rheumatol. 1999;18:264–5.
20. Charalambous CP, Tryfonidis S, Sadiq P, et al. Septic arthritis following intra-articular steroid injection of the knee: a survey of current practice regarding antiseptic technique used during intra-articular steroid injection of the knee. Clin Rheumatol. 2003;22:386–90.
21. Lazarevic MB, Skosey JL, Djordjevic-Denic G, et al. Reduction of cortisol levels after single-intra-articular and intramuscular steroid injection. Am J Med. 1995;99:370–3.
22. Godwin M, Dawes M. Intra-articular steroid injections for painful knees: systematic review with meta-analysis. Can Fam Physician. 2004;50:241–8.
23. Slotkoff AT, Clauw DJ, Nashel DJ. Effect of soft tissue corticosteroid injection on glucose control in diabetics. Arthritis Rheum. 1994;37:S347 (abstract).
24. Nesbitt LT. Minimizing complications from systemic glucocorticosteroid use. Clin Dermatol. 1995;13:925–39.
25. Gensler L. Glucocorticoids: complications to anticipate and prevent. Neurohospitalist. 2012;3:92–7.
26. Emkey RD, Lindsay R, Lissy J, et al. The systemic effect of intraarticular administration of corticosteroid on markers of bone formation and bone formation and bone resorption in patients with rheumatoid arthritis. Arthritis Rheum. 1996;39:277–82.
27. Moreland L, O'Dell J. Glucocorticoids in rheumatoid arthritis. Arthritis Rheum. 2002;46:2553–63.
28. afKlint E, Grundman C, Engström M, et al. Intra-articular glucocorticoid treatment reduces inflammation in synovial cell infiltrations more efficiently than in synovial cell infiltrations more efficiently than in synovial blood vessels. Arthritis Rheum. 2005;52:3880–9.
29. Neeli I, Khan SN, Radic M. Histone deimination as a response to inflammatory stimuli in neutrophils. J Immunol. 2008;180:1895–902.
30. Makrygiannakis D, Revu S, Engström M, et al. Local administration of glucocorticoids decreases synovial citrullination in rheumatoid arthritis. Arthritis Res Ther. 2012;14:1–9.
31. Chatham W, Williams G, Moreland L, et al. Intraarticular corticosteroid injections: should we rest the joints? Arthritis Care Res. 1989;2:70–4.

32. Boesen M, Boesen L, Jensen KE, et al. Clinical outcome and imaging changes after intraarticular (IA) application of etanercept or methylprednisolone in rheumatoid arthritis: magnetic resonance imaging and ultrasound-Doppler show no effect on IA injections in the wrist after 4 weeks. J Rheumatol. 2008;35:584–91.
33. Hertzberger-Ten RC, deVries-van der Vluge BLM, et al. Intra-articular steroids in pauciarticular juvenile chronic arthritis, type 1. Eur J Pediatr. 1991;150:170–2.
34. Bloom B, Alaria A, Miller L. Intra-articular corticosteroid therapy for juvenile idiopathic arthritis: report of an experiential cohort and literature review. Rheumatol Int. 2011;31: 749–56.
35. Beukelman T, Guevara JP, Albert DA. Optimal treatment of knee monoarthritis in juvenile idiopathic arthritis: a decision analysis. Arthritis Rheum. 2008;59:1580–8.
36. Lepore L, del Santo M, Malargio C, et al. Treatment of juvenile idiopathic arthritis with intraarticular triamcinolone hexacetonide: evaluation of clinical effectiveness correlated with ANA and T gamma/delta+ and B CD5+ lymphocyte populations of synovial fluid. Clin Exp Rheumatol. 2002;20:719–22.
37. Huppertz HI, Tschammler A, Horwitz AE, et al. Intraarticular corticosteroids for chronic arthritis in children: efficacy and effects on cartilage and growth. J Pediatr. 1995;127:317–21.
38. Zulian F, Martini G, Gobber D, et al. Triamcinolone acetonide and hexacetonide intraarticular treatment of symmetrical joints in juvenile idiopathic arthritis: a double blind trial. Rheumatology (Oxford). 2004;43:1288–91.
39. Gran JT, Husby G. Ankylosing spondylitis. Current drug treatment. Drugs. 1992;44: 585–603.
40. Gunaydin I, Pereira PL, Fritz J, et al. Magnetic resonance imaging guided corticosteroid injection of sacroiliac joints in patients with spondylarthropathy. Are multiple injections more beneficial? Rheumatol Int. 2006;26:396–400.
41. Braun J, van den Berg R, Baraliokos X, et al. Computed tomography guided corticosteroid injection of the sacroiliac joint in patients with spondyloarthropathy with sacroiliitis: clinical outcome and follow up by dynamic magnetic resonance imaging. J Rheumatol. 1996;23: 659–64.
42. Spies CM, Burmester GR, Buttgereit F. Analysis of similarities and differences in glucocorticoid therapy between rheumatoid arthritis and ankylosing spondylitis – a systemic comparison. Clin Exp Rheumat. 2009;27 Suppl 55:S152–8.
43. Wechalekar M, Vinik O, Schlesinger M, et al. Intra-articular glucocorticoids for acute gout. Cochrane Database Syst Rev. 2013;(4):1–16.
44. Richette P, Pardin T. Gout. Lancet. 2010;375(9711):318–28.
45. Koski JM. Ultrasound guided injection in rheumatology. J Rheumatol. 2000;27:2131–8.
46. Balint PV, Kane D, Hunter J, et al. Ultrasound guided versus conventional joint and soft tissue fluid aspiration in rheumatology practice: a pilot study. J Rheumatol. 2002;29:2209–13.
47. Sibbitt WL, Peisajovich A, Michael AA, et al. Does sonographic needle guidance affect the clinical outcome of intraarticular injections? J Rheumatol. 2009;36:1892–902.
48. Raza K, Lee CY, Pilling D, et al. Ultrasound guidance allows accurate needle placement and aspiration from small joints in patients with early inflammatory arthritis. Rheumatology. 2003;42:976–9.
49. Brostrom E, Hagelber S, Haglund-Akerlind Y. Effect of joint injections in children with juvenile idiopathic arthritis: evaluation by 3D-gait analysis. Acta Paediatr. 2004;93:906–10.

NSAIDs

4

Wolfgang W. Bolten

Contents

4.1   Nonsteroidal Anti-inflammatory Drugs

4.1.1   Efficacy and Tolerability

Nonsteroidal anti-inflammatory drugs (NSAIDs) are the most favorite drugs for the treatment of somatoform pain in osteoarthritis, rheumatoid arthritis, psoriatic arthritis, or pain associated with other arthritides from unknown origin, as well as peripheral and axial spondyloarthritides. Thus, NSAIDs cover the entire area of the treatment of inflammatory pain in musculoskeletal disorders [1]. Regarding their effectiveness NSAIDs surpass other analgesics including opioids. Comparing the mean efficacy of different NSAIDs, no relevant differences can be found if the

W.W. Bolten
Rheumatologie, Praxis Dr. von Seck, Rheinstrasse 31, Wiesbaden 65185, Germany

Rheumatologie, Klaus-Miehlke Klinik Wiesbaden, Leibnizstraße 23,
Wiesbaden 65191, Germany
e-mail: wbolten@em.uni-frankfurt.de

© Springer International Publishing Switzerland 2015
W.U. Kampen, M. Fischer (eds.), *Local Treatment of Inflammatory Joint Diseases: Benefits and Risks*, DOI 10.1007/978-3-319-16949-1_4

approved maximum daily dose is used for each NSAID. However, from the perspective of an individual patient, the effectiveness of different NSAIDs differs widely. Thus, the change to a different NSAID in case of insufficient pain relief still may reach the therapeutic goal.

Because of the frequent use of NSAIDs, their spectrum of side effects is well known. Among </=65-year old and otherwise healthy patients with rheumatic pain, clinically relevant side effects belong to the rare events. Thus, prophylactic therapeutic interventions or routine monitoring for prevention of serious adverse effects in this patient group is not necessary, and therapy costs remain to be low.

However in about 15 % up to 40 % of patients, the NSAID therapy interferes with heartburn, dyspeptic complaints, nausea, or abdominal pain without any endoscopically proven severe gastrointestinal lesions. Proton pump inhibitors are recommended for the treatment of dyspeptic complaints. Changing the NSAID may also be a good choice in this clinical setting. Regardless of the symptomatic efficacy of the therapy, 10 % of patients with GI complaints discontinue the NSAID treatment.

4.1.2 Increased Intolerance in Patients at Risk

Common patients suffering from painful musculoskeletal disease, particularly from arthrosis of the large joints, are older patients >65 years in daily clinical practice. The average effectiveness of NSAIDs is also satisfying. But with increasing age, the rate of clinically significant side effects rises. Among the most serious adverse events, gastrointestinal mucosal defects, impairment of renal function, and – more frequently analyzed in the last few years – cardiovascular damage dominate the scientific discussion. In addition to the higher age, other risk factors emerged from postmarketing clinical trials. If individual risk profiles are considered, appropriate preventive measures can be done to monitor and improve the safety of the patient.

4.1.3 Gastrointestinal Side Effects

Important and meaningful risk indicators for increased gastrointestinal (GI) risk are GI diseases (e.g., history of a GI ulcer), higher age (>60–65 years old), severe concomitant diseases, and comedication with glucocorticoids, anticoagulants, or antidepressants from the type of selective serotonin/serotonin noradrenalin reuptake inhibitors (SSRI/SSNRI) which emerged [2]. Important GI risk indicators are listed in Table 4.1. Helicobacter pylori infection increases the risk of ulcer regardless of the therapy with traditional NSAIDs [3]. Similarly, nicotine and alcohol consumption act as independent risk factors and affect the GI tract regardless of the NSAID therapy.

Upper gastrointestinal ulceration, bleeding, and perforation are the most frequent serious, life-threatening NSAID side effects. They occur in 1–2 % of patients under long-term treatment with traditional NSAIDs, in about half of the cases without any preceding clinical alarming symptoms. Under regular intake of NSAID, the GI risk

Table 4.1 Gastrointestinal risk indicators

High NSAID dose
Age (60 to) 65 years of age or older
History of gastroduodenal ulcer, GI bleeding, or gastrointestinal perforation
Adjuvant treatment with anticoagulants, platelet aggregation inhibitors, glucocorticoids, or antidepressants (SSRIS and SSNRI[a])
Severe comorbidity, such as cardiovascular disease, heart failure, liver or kidney functional impairment (including dehydration), diabetes mellitus, hypertension
Long-term needs of a NSAID therapy (e.g., spondyloarthritis, rheumatoid arthritis, or osteoarthritis or chronic low-back pain in patients over 45 years)

[a]Selective serotonin/serotonin noradrenalin reuptake inhibitors

increases by a factor 2–4. The mortality rate is 10–15 %. Of 1,200 patients treated with traditional NSAIDs for more than 2 months, one dies due to the associated GI complications [4].

The lower GI tract is less well studied. Occult chronic bleeding in the small intestine or colon is lately recognized by worsening of an anemia [5]. In patients with inflammatory bowel diseases (e.g., Crohn, ulcerative colitis), an exacerbation threatens during treatment with traditional NSAIDs.

GI risk remains unchanged during the entire course of the NSAID therapy [6]. They will not occur during discontinuations of therapy and not after cessation of NSAID treatment [7, 8]. However, there are no meaningful data from studies with an observation period longer than 1 year [6].

4.1.4 Cardiovascular Side Effects

Vascular events such as myocardial infarction, stroke, or fatal cardiovascular complications occur about three times more often in patients with NSAIDs than in patients without NSAID medication. This significant increase was statistically proven in large clinical trials and meta-analyses for coxibs and diclofenac. An increase of the coronary risk could be shown for higher-dosed ibuprofen (1,200 mg/day) (RR 2.22; $p = 0.0253$). A similar high cardiovascular (CV) risk can be assumed for other less-investigated NSAIDs. High-dosed naproxen as an exception behaves neutral in terms of CV risk (RR 0.93). Low-dose ibuprofen does not increase the thromboembolic CV event rates. With all NSAIDs the risk of severe heart failure is doubled [6]. Increase in blood pressure is more common in patients taking etoricoxib than others taking naproxen or ibuprofen. In several observational studies, rofecoxib, celecoxib, and diclofenac dose dependently increased the risk of vascular adverse drug reactions by 20–30 % [6, 9]. One year of NSAID treatment with 1,000 patients at moderate CV risk results in three additional clinically relevant CV events including one fatal event [6, 7].

The common CV risk factors (e.g., hypertension, diabetes mellitus, hyperlipidemia, smoking, a history of CV disease such as coronary heart disease or myocardial infarction, positive family history with CV disease in ≤50-year-old patients) also apply to NSAID patients as predictors of increased CV risk; also the average risk increases with the NSAID dose and the duration of treatment [10]. But even without a corresponding risk factor, the rate of NSAID-associated CV side effects is slightly increased [6, 11–13]. Especially the risk of severe heart failure under any NSAID therapy is doubled independently of the platelet function [6]. Other studies have found an increased risk of stroke. However, the data in this area are not sufficient for a final assessment. Even after many years of NSAID treatment, an adaption of risk cannot be observed. After cessation of NSAIDs, the individual risk quickly disappears [10].

The FDA alerts of an increased CV risk in any NSAID therapy. In patients with coronary heart disease or congestive heart failure (NYHA grade ≥2) or history of stroke, the EMA declares the coxibs and diclofenac as contraindicated. With any NSAID therapy in patients at CV risk, the EMA urges caution [14].

CV and GI risks often are increased at the same time, especially in elderly patients. In patients with moderate combined CV and GI risks, vascular or gastrointestinal complications are expected to occur in 4–19 % [7] after a 10-year high-dose NSAID therapy.

4.1.5 The Renovascular Risk

Several physiological products of the COX enzymes are significantly involved in the regulation of renal function. NSAIDs interfere with the COX-1- and COX-2-dependent renal tissue level of prostaglandins. During the first 30 days of NSAID treatment, elderly patients (>65 years) have a significantly increased risk of acute renal failure (RR: 2.05. [15]), and a NSAID therapy lowers the glomerular filtration rate in patients with chronic kidney disease [16]. The risk of hypertension is increased [17–20]. In damaged kidneys water retention and edema are common events.

Other manifestations of diseases and serious side effects (liver, skin, etc.) are possible but occur rarely.

4.1.6 Mechanism of Action

All NSAIDs inhibit the enzyme cyclooxygenase (COX) which interferes with the paracrine synthesis of prostaglandins (PGs) [21]. Prostaglandins regulate specific physiological processes via two different COX enzymes, dependent on the tissue location. COX-2 is induced in injured tissues. This isoenzyme synthesizes PGs, which locally induce inflammatory processes and mediate pain.

In other tissues, prostaglandins are synthesized continuously. This is especially important in the GI tract whose mucosa constantly expresses COX-1 and produces PGs to protect the tissue against low pH levels. Traditional NSAIDs (tNSAIDs) inhibit both isoenzymes of cyclooxygenases. Desired effects (pain relief through inhibition of COX-2-specific PG synthesis), as well as adverse effects (mucosa lesions due to elimination of the COX-1-mediated protective PGs), are attributed to the same principle, the inhibition of the synthesis of PGs. Individual effect and side-effect differences result from differences in organ tissue and metabolic reactions.

In therapeutic doses, selective COX-2 inhibitors (coxibs) virtually do not react with the COX-1, and therefore the gastrointestinal toxicity of coxibs is less than that of tNSAIDs [22].

NSAIDs usually are administered orally and are absorbed in the intestine. Thus, their effect is systemically mediated. This is true for the inflamed articular tissue as well as for the gastrointestinal tract. Some NSAIDs undergo an enterohepatic cycle and pass multiple times through the small intestine. In this case an additional local potential of harm could be added to the systemic toxicity.

Parenteral routes of administration have no advantage related to the gastrointestinal potential danger but bear greater local risks. Thus, this kind of application should be avoided. Suppositories have a longer residence time in the rectum, and therefore, local toxic effects cannot be ruled out. On the other hand, they are frequently eliminated in advance via naturalis, or they are insufficiently absorbed. That is why suppositories do not provide benefits in clinical trials, and therefore they are not recommended for pain therapy [23, 24].

Topical NSAIDs – containing ointments, gels, solutions, or patches, applied on the intact skin – alleviate musculoskeletal pain better than placebo [25] and are not inferior compared to oral NSAIDs therapy [25–27]. Their mode of action is unclear. Thus, topical NSAIDs can be used tentatively as low-risk NSAID preparation.

4.1.7 Prophylactic Aspects

The risk of GI complications can be reduced by 50 % if a coxib instead of a tNSAID is used. An equally effective approach is to use a proton pump inhibitor (PPI) or misoprostol accompanying the intake of a NSAID. The PPI protects the gastroduodenal part of the GI tract but not the lower GI tract; misoprostol in turn has a higher potential for adverse GI symptoms. In high-risk patients where NSAID therapy is planned to be resumed despite an occurred GI complication, a treatment strategy with a coxib in combination with a PPI is recommended, thus avoiding recurrence of ulcers.

Naproxen should be the first choice in patients with higher CV risk requiring high doses of NSAID because of its CV-neutral action. Patients with increased GI and CV risks at the same time should also use naproxen (to cover low NSAID need instead of naproxen, low-dose ibuprofen is recommended) in combination with PPI. In case of a comedication with low-dose aspirin, one has to consider that the cardioprotective effect of aspirin can be limited via interaction with tNSAID particularly ibuprofen competing at the COX-1 receptor.

Patients with mild-to-moderate renal impairment (GFR 30–60 ml/min) and urgent NSAID demand should be treated with reduced NSAID dose, and periodical test of renal function is recommended. NSAID therapy is no longer recommended below a GFR of 30 ml/min. In any case the NSAID dose has to be chosen as low as reasonably practicable, and the benefits of additional physical treatment have to be exhausted.

If NSAID therapy is not effective or contraindicated, other pharmacological approaches (glucocorticoids, analgesics) have to be considered. Patients with mono- or oligoarthritis without permanent pain relief despite exhausted pharmacological therapy potentially benefit from surgical or radiation synovectomy.

References

1. Mutschler E, Geisslinger G, Kroemer HK, Menzel S, Ruth P. Mutschler Arzneimittelwirkungen: Pharmakologie – Klinische Pharmakologie – Toxikologie. 9th ed. Stuttgart: Wissenschaftliche Verlagsgesellschaft; 2012.
2. Vandraas KF, Spigset O, Mahic M, Slordal L. Non-steroidal anti-inflammatory drugs: use and co-treatment with potentially interacting medications in the elderly. Eur J Clin Pharmacol. 2010;66(8):823–9. PubMed Epub 2010/04/21. eng.
3. Tielemans MM, Eikendal T, Jansen JB, van Oijen MG. Identification of NSAID users at risk for gastrointestinal complications: a systematic review of current guidelines and consensus agreements. Drug Saf. 2010;33(6):443–53. PubMed Epub 2010/05/22. eng.
4. Tramer MR, Moore RA, Reynolds DJ, McQuay HJ. Quantitative estimation of rare adverse events which follow a biological progression: a new model applied to chronic NSAID use. Pain. 2000;85(1-2):169–82. PubMed.
5. Chan FK, Lanas A, Scheiman J, Berger MF, Nguyen H, Goldstein JL. Celecoxib versus omeprazole and diclofenac in patients with osteoarthritis and rheumatoid arthritis (CONDOR): a randomised trial. Lancet. 2010;376(9736):173–9. PubMed Epub 2010/07/20. eng.
6. Coxib and traditional NSAID Trialists' (CNT) Collaboration. Vascular and upper gastrointestinal effects of non-steroidal anti-inflammatory drugs: meta-analyses of individual participant data from randomised trials. Lancet. 2013;382(9894):769–79.
7. Griffin MR. High-dose non-steroidal anti-inflammatories: painful choices. Lancet. 2013; 382(9894):746–8. PubMed NSAID!.
8. Hernandez-Diaz S, Rodriguez LA. Association between nonsteroidal anti-inflammatory drugs and upper gastrointestinal tract bleeding/perforation: an overview of epidemiologic studies published in the 1990s. Arch Intern Med. 2000;160(14):2093–9. PubMed Epub 2000/07/25. eng.
9. McGettigan P, Henry D. Cardiovascular risk with non-steroidal anti-inflammatory drugs: systematic review of population-based controlled observational studies. PLoS Med. 2011; 8(9):e1001098. PubMed Pubmed Central PMCID: PMC3181230. Epub 2011/10/08. eng.
10. García Rodríguez LA, Tacconelli S, Patrignani P. Role of dose potency in the prediction of risk of myocardial infarction associated with nonsteroidal anti-inflammatory drugs in the general population. J Am Coll Cardiol. 2008;52(20):1628–36.
11. Fosbol EL, Gislason GH, Jacobsen S, Folke F, Hansen ML, Schramm TK, et al. Risk of myocardial infarction and death associated with the use of nonsteroidal anti-inflammatory drugs (NSAIDs) among healthy individuals: a nationwide cohort study. Clin Pharmacol Ther. 2009;85(2):190–7. PubMed Epub 2008/11/07. eng.
12. McGettigan P, Henry D. Use of non-steroidal anti-inflammatory drugs that elevate cardiovascular risk: an examination of sales and essential medicines lists in low-, middle-, and high-income countries. PLoS Med. 2013;10(2):e1001388. PubMed Pubmed Central PMCID: 3570554.
13. Gislason GH, Jacobsen S, Rasmussen JN, Rasmussen S, Buch P, Friberg J, et al. Risk of death or reinfarction associated with the use of selective cyclooxygenase-2 inhibitors and nonselective nonsteroidal antiinflammatory drugs after acute myocardial infarction. Circulation. 2006;113(25):2906–13. PubMed Epub 2006/06/21. eng.

14. EMA. European Medicines Agency concludes action on COX-2 inhibitors. European Medicines Agency [Internet]. 2005; (Doc. Ref. EMEA/207766/2005). Available from: http://www.ema.europa.eu/ema/index.jsp?curl=pages/news_and_events/news/2010/01/news_detail_000969.jsp&mid=WC0b01ac058004d5c1.

15. Schneider V, Levesque LE, Zhang B, Hutchinson T, Brophy JM. Association of selective and conventional nonsteroidal antiinflammatory drugs with acute renal failure: A population-based, nested case-control analysis. Am J Epidemiol. 2006;164(9):881–9. PubMed Epub 2006/09/29. eng.

16. Gooch K, Culleton BF, Manns BJ, Zhang J, Alfonso H, Tonelli M, et al. NSAID use and progression of chronic kidney disease. Am J Med. 2007;120(3):280e1–7. PubMed Epub 2007/03/14. eng.

17. Aw TJ, Haas SJ, Liew D, Krum H. Meta-analysis of cyclooxygenase-2 inhibitors and their effects on blood pressure. Arch Intern Med. 2005;165(5):490–6. PubMed Epub 2005/02/16. eng.

18. Zhang J, Ding EL, Song Y. Adverse effects of cyclooxygenase 2 inhibitors on renal and arrhythmia events: meta-analysis of randomized trials. JAMA. 2006;296(13):1619–32. PubMed Epub 2006/09/14. eng.

19. Morrison A, Ramey DR, van Adelsberg J, Watson DJ. Systematic review of trials of the effect of continued use of oral non-selective NSAIDs on blood pressure and hypertension. Curr Med Res Opin. 2007;23(10):2395–404. PubMed.

20. Chan CC, Reid CM, Aw TJ, Liew D, Haas SJ, Krum H. Do COX-2 inhibitors raise blood pressure more than nonselective NSAIDs and placebo? An updated meta-analysis. J Hypertens. 2009;27(12):2332–41. PubMed Epub 2009/11/06. eng.

21. Vane JR. Inhibition of prostaglandin synthesis as a mechanism of action for aspirin-like drugs. Nat New Biol. 1971;231(25):232–5. PubMed.

22. Bombardier C. An evidence-based evaluation of the gastrointestinal safety of coxibs. Am J Cardiol. 2002;89(6A):3D–9. PubMed Epub 2002/03/23. eng.

23. Fortun PJ, Hawkey CJ. Nonsteroidal antiinflammatory drugs and the small intestine. Curr Opin Gastroenterol. 2007;23(2):134–41. PubMed Epub 2007/02/03. eng.

24. Tramer MR, Williams JE, Carroll D, Wiffen PJ, Moore RA, McQuay HJ. Comparing analgesic efficacy of non-steroidal anti-inflammatory drugs given by different routes in acute and chronic pain: a qualitative systematic review. Acta Anaesthesiol Scand. 1998;42(1):71–9. PubMed.

25. Moore RA, Derry S, McQuay HJ. Topical agents in the treatment of rheumatic pain. Rheum Dis Clin North Am. 2008;34(2):415–32. PubMed Epub 2008/07/22. eng.

26. Derry S, Moore RA, Rabbie R. Topical NSAIDs for chronic musculoskeletal pain in adults. Cochrane Database Syst Rev. 2012;(9):CD007400-CD. PubMed PMID: MEDLINE:22972108.

27. Conaghan PG, Dickson J, Bolten W, Cevc G, Rother M. A multicentre, randomized, placebo- and active-controlled trial comparing the efficacy and safety of topical ketoprofen in transfersome gel (IDEA-033) with ketoprofen-free vehicle (TDT 064) and oral celecoxib for knee pain associated with osteoarthritis. Rheumatology (Oxford). 2013;52(7):1303–12. PubMed.

Synovectomy of Rheumatoid Joints

5

Josef Zacher

Contents

5.1 Introduction

Rheumatoid arthritis (RA) like similar other inflammatory joint diseases is an auto-immune disease targeting also the synovial lining of all joints. Synovitis and pannus formation may actively destruct articular cartilage and subchondral bone if untreated (Fig. 5.1). During the last three decades, the development of new medical treatments especially the so-called biologicals alone or in combination with standard disease-modifying antirheumatic drugs made enormous progress in controlling the inflammatory and destructive process. Despite this there are still patients with chronic synovitis of their joints and progression of destruction.

Surgical removal of all macroscopic detectable inflamed synovial tissue – synovectomy – is an established method of treatment for longer-lasting synovitis for rheumatoid patients complaining of joint swelling, tenderness, and pain despite

J. Zacher
Centre of Orthopedic and Trauma Surgery, HELIOS Klinikum Berlin Buch,
Schwanebecker Chaussee 50, 13125 Berlin, Germany
e-mail: josef.zacher@helios-kliniken.de

© Springer International Publishing Switzerland 2015
W.U. Kampen, M. Fischer (eds.), *Local Treatment of Inflammatory Joint
Diseases: Benefits and Risks*, DOI 10.1007/978-3-319-16949-1_5

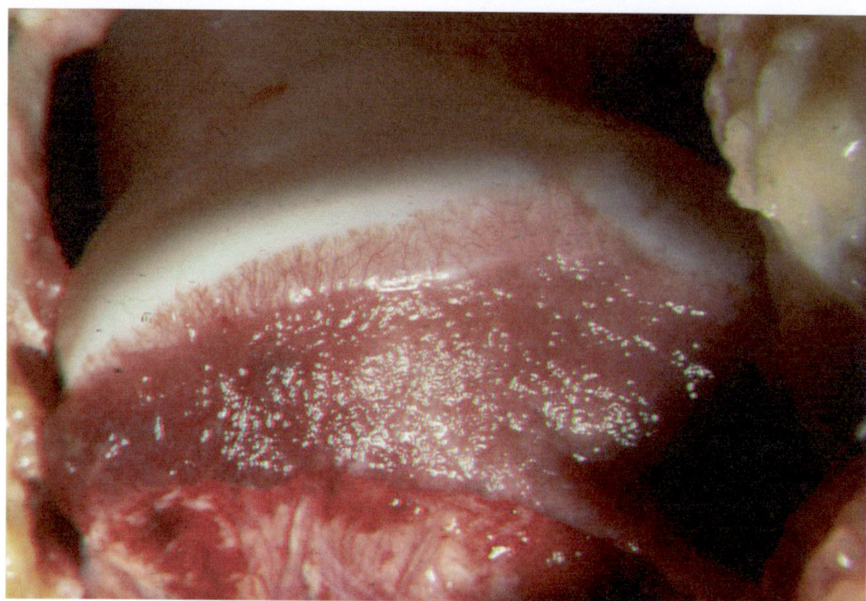

Fig. 5.1 Synovitis and pannus growing over the articular cartilage at the lateral femur condyle in a patient with rheumatoid arthritis of the knee

Table 5.1 Larsen's grading system for RA

Grade	Definition
0	Normal
1	Soft tissue swelling, slight joint space narrowing (<25 % of the original joint space), periarticular osteoporosis
2	Definite early abnormality, one or several small erosions
3	Medium destructive abnormality, marked erosions
4	Severe destructive abnormality, large erosions
5	Gross deformity, the bony outlines of the joint have disappeared

regular medical therapy for 6 months. The exact timing for surgical intervention should be the result of an interdisciplinary discussion between internal and orthopedic rheumatologist.

Synovitis in osteoarthritis in contrast to rheumatic diseases is a cytokine-dependent reaction to detritus originating from cartilage breakdown. The rationale to remove synovitis by surgical means does not work in osteoarthritis because the underlying disease is the problem of cartilage breakdown which is not addressed by synovectomy. Synovectomy in osteoarthritic conditions has shown little short-lasting benefit and overall disappointing clinical outcomes and therefore is not recommended in recent guidelines.

Early synovectomy is performed in radiological Larsen stages 0-II, late synovectomy in Larsen stages III-IV (Table 5.1). It is thought that an early synovectomy may prevent further joint destruction but clinical trials of high quality to prove this are lacking. Late synovectomies have the goal to decrease pain and improve function.

At present there are no comparative clinical data for a staged algorithm if synovectomy or radiosynoviorthesis should be performed first or which intervention is superior to the other. RSO may be preferred as it is less invasive needing no systemic anesthesia. RSO can be repeated and has the possibility of open surgery if being not successful. On the other hand there are hints that synovectomy closely followed by RSO may lead to better outcomes in knee synovectomy. Further controlled trials are needed.

As a result of the tremendous progress in medical treatment, the need for surgical interventions in arthritic joints declined over the last three decades in many countries. Especially the numbers of synovectomy dropped steadily also in Germany from a reported 5.6 % of rheumatoid patients in 1993 to 3.5 % in 2000 to 0.3 % in 2008 [1].

5.2   Synovectomy of the Knee

As synovectomies of the knee are the most common interventions, there are more data about results of treatment available than in other joints.

Synovectomy of the knee may be performed as an arthroscopic or open surgery. Arthroscopic synovectomy is mostly performed in early Larsen stages and demonstrated its effectivity in a multicenter trial of 93 knee joints in 81 patients with early forms of rheumatoid arthritis at a follow-up time of 33 months [2]. The Lysholm score (an established knee score relating to pain, swelling, instability, and functional outcome: 0–100 points) increased from 43.2 points preoperatively to 78.1 points. The Insall knee and functional score (an established knee score especially for use in knee joint replacement relating to pain and range of motion, 100 points, and additionally to knee function, 100 points) showed a highly significant increase of 25.7 and 25.2 points to 71.2 and 80.2 points, respectively. Among the individual variables investigated, pain, swelling, and walking distance in particular were improved. Larsen stages worsened slightly from 1.57 preoperatively to 1.95 at follow-up.

Even in advanced Larsen stages, open synovectomy of the knee demonstrated over a period of more than 10 years (10.1; range 6.4–12.7) a long-lasting improvement of function [3]. Despite reasonable functional results radiographic progression of disease was observed (Larsen stage 2.2–3.7). The need for joint replacement in nearly three-quarters of the patients could be delayed for more than 10 years.

A recent meta-analysis [4] analyzed all published synovectomy trials to find out whether open or arthroscopic surgery leads to better results. Arthroscopic and open synovectomy provided similar pain relief (Fig. 5.2a) at last follow-up for knees ($p = 0.16$).

Arthroscopic synovectomy was more likely than open synovectomy to lead to recurrence of synovitis at knees ($p < 0.001$) and to lead to radiographic progression (Fig. 5.2b) for knees ($p = 0.001$). Open synovectomies were more likely to require

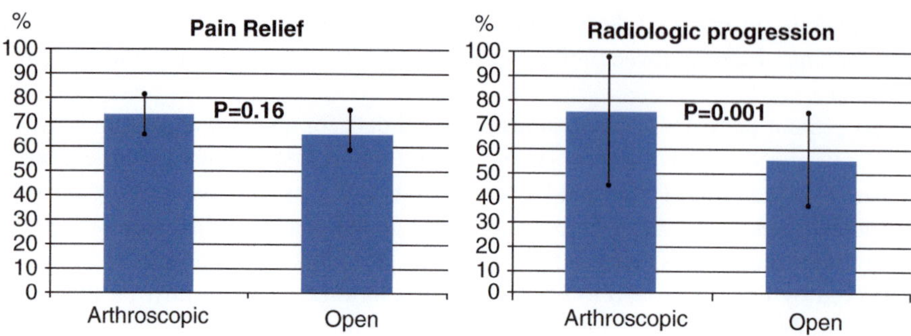

Fig. 5.2 Mean results after synovectomy of the knee. (**a**) Percentage of patients with pain relief. (**b**) Percentage of patients with radiologic progression [4]

joint replacement or arthrodesis ($p=0.01$) at last follow-up, but this may be influenced by an indication bias as the number of patients with advanced rheumatoid arthritis at time of intervention was nearly double as high in open synovectomy.

In the multicenter trial with a mean follow-up of 33 months [2], patients receiving additional radiation synovectomy showed a highly significantly better result than those receiving synovectomy alone. In contrast to this finding, this positive effect does not seem to last over time as in a 14-year follow-up trial, it was found that after 5 years there was a steadily increase in worsening of joint destruction leading to joint replacement. Nearly half of the knees were converted to joint replacement after 10 years and 60.4 % after 14 years. This observation challenges the long-term benefit of the combined procedure.

5.3 Synovectomy of the Hip

There have been disappointing results in cases of synovectomy of the hip joint in adults especially in late-stage cases. Therefore, it is not recommended as a standard procedure at time although clinical trials are lacking. It seems to be more promising to perform total joint replacement in advanced stages of rheumatoid hip involvement instead.

There are data in patients with juvenile arthritis showing that even in late stages of the disease (Larsen III and higher) open synovectomy combined with soft tissue procedures leads to an improvement in function [6]. Merle d'Aubigné hip score (an established hip score relating to pain, range of motion, and walking ability: 0–18 points) significantly improved from 9.5 ± 2.5 points at baseline to 16.3 ± 1.0 points at the time of follow-up ($p<0.001$). The individual scores for pain, mobility, and walking ability were significantly increased as well (all $p<0.001$). Eighty-five percent of the 56 hips were observed to have a very great or great improvement in function. Osteonecrosis of the femoral head was not observed. Five hips required total hip arthroplasty during the follow-up period. Thus, the survival rate for the hips was 94 % at a mean of 4 years following the synovectomy.

5.4 Synovectomy of the Ankle Joint

Open synovectomies in the ankle joint may still be the standard of care as in more than 90 % of the patients additional surgical procedures at tendons have to be performed. Arthroscopic synovectomies may be performed in isolated ankle joint involvement.

An observation trial [7] showed a significant, but clinically moderate, gain in the Kofoed ankle score (a score established for evaluation in ankle arthroplasty: 50 points for pain, 20 for range of motion, and 30 for ankle function) from 42.4 to 55.9 points ($p = 0.042$), which was mainly caused by pain reduction and gain of mobility, whereas a decline of function was detected. Pain (VAS) decreased from 7.6 to 3.3 ($p < 0.001$) and 81.5 % of the patients assessed the results of the synovectomy as good or very good. But as in other joints, progression of the Larsen grade was found in 62 % of the ankle joints.

5.5 Synovectomy of the Shoulder

In the natural course of rheumatoid arthritis, the shoulder joint is affected in most of the patients. Synovitis not only leads to pain and lack of function of the glenohumeral joint but also destroys tendon structures (rotator cuff, long head of the biceps tendon) and causes subacromial bursitis.

There is only little evidence of outcome after open surgical interventions. But case series clearly showed pain relief in 80–100 % for at least 5–8 years despite some worsening in radiological Larsen score over time.

Arthroscopic synovectomy may be suitable in uncomplicated cases, but if any major tears of the rotator cuff have to be treated, a mini open access allows better visibility. Refixation of the rotator cuff to bone with suture anchors may be compromised by poor bone stock. Suture technique has to be adjusted [8].

One case series [9] in patients with synovitis of the glenohumeral joint and no affection to the rotator cuff showed an improvement in pain at a mean follow-up of 5.5 years in 13 of 16 patients ($P < 0.001$). The results regarding improvements in range of motion were less predictable. Seven of eight shoulders followed-up radiographically for more than 1 year showed radiographic progression of disease.

5.6 Synovectomy of the Elbow

About half of the rheumatoid patients have an involvement of the elbow joint after 15 years of disease duration. Synovitis of the elbow early decreases the range of motion regarding supination/pronation and an extension lag occurs. In later stages also flexion beyond 90° will be lost.

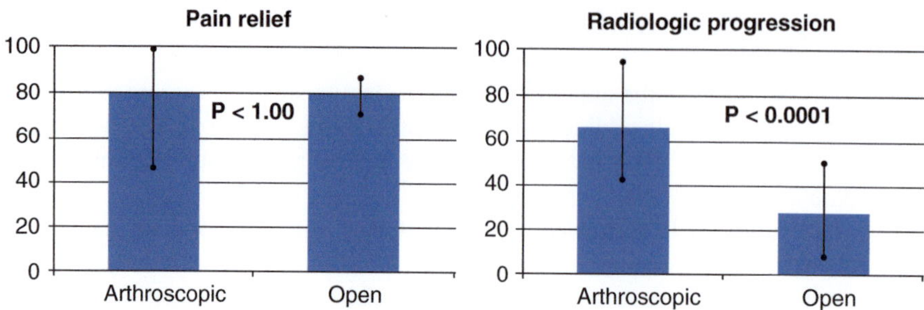

Fig. 5.3 Mean results after synovectomy of the elbow. (**a**) Percentage of patients with pain relief. (**b**) Percentage of patients with radiologic progression [4]

Open surgery is well established and allows a very extensive completeness of synovectomy. Elbow arthroscopy is known as a technically challenging procedure and bears the potential risk of nerve injuries.

A recent meta-analysis [4] analyzed all published synovectomy trials to find out whether open or arthroscopic surgery leads to better results. Arthroscopic and open synovectomy provided similar pain relief (Fig. 5.3a) at last follow-up for elbows (79.4±31.1 % vs. 80.0±9.7 %; $p = 1.00$).

Arthroscopic synovectomy was more likely than open synovectomy to lead to recurrence of synovitis for elbows (21.9±7.9 % vs. 9.3±8.9 %; $p = 0.03$) and to lead to radiographic progression (Fig. 5.3b) for elbows (65.6±29.9 % vs. 27.7±22.7 %; $p < 0.001$). Both interventions were equally likely to require subsequent arthroplasty in elbows ($p = 0.91$).

Similar results were observed in a case series of open and arthroscopic interventions in Japan [10] and South Korea [11].

5.7 Synovectomy of the Wrist

Wrist involvement is very common in rheumatoid arthritis: about 40 % during the first 2 years up to 90 % in the long term [12]. During the natural course of the disease in most patients, there is not only an isolated involvement of the wrist, but also the tendons are affected by tenosynovitis.

Thus, the surgical intervention mostly cares for both: synovitis and tenosynovitis. Results of case series up to 10 years after intervention showed an increased range of motion, improvement of pain and function at follow-up, but also a marked worsening of the radiological Larsen stage at the wrist.

Arthroscopic synovectomy is a well-accepted method in early stage rheumatoid arthritis (RA), but its use is controversial in advanced RA of the wrist [13]. The results of a small case series showed pain relief, improvement in function, but no improvement in range of motion or grip strength.

Overall early synovectomies at the rheumatoid wrist may delay further complex surgery as wrist arthrodesis or wrist arthroplasty.

5.8   Synovectomy of Finger Joints

Finger joints are typically involved at any stages in the course of rheumatoid arthritis, especially all metacarpophalangeal (MCP) and the proximal interphalangeal (PIP) joints. Chronic synovitis at these joints not only leads to destruction of cartilage and bone but also to a distension of the capsule and a dealignment of tendons causing typical deformities like 90/90 deformity of the thumb MCP joint or boutonniere deformity of the PIP joints (Fig. 5.4).

If synovitis is accompanied by one of these deformities, open synovectomy is the standard of care to address the pathology of the synovium and the deformity of the tendons and capsule. There is only limited evidence about the outcome regarding pain, function, or radiological progress of the rheumatoid disease.

As arthroscopic instruments for small joints improved and surgical experience grows, also the small joint of the fingers were addressed by arthroscope for synovectomy [14, 15]. Because the PIP joint space was not wide enough to insert the arthroscope into the palmar cavity, the palmar part of the articular surfaces and the volar synovium could not be inspected.

Short-term (12-month) results and patient satisfaction have been quoted excellent.

5.9   Surgical Complications After Synovectomy

Little data from prospective trials are available about surgical complications of synovectomies in different joints. In one prospective study in 201 patients [16], complications after arthroscopic synovectomy of the knee included septic arthritis (0.5 %), superficial wound healing problems (2 %), and intraarticular hematoma (3.5 %). Complete recovery was achieved after complications were treated, and the result of the synovectomy was not compromised.

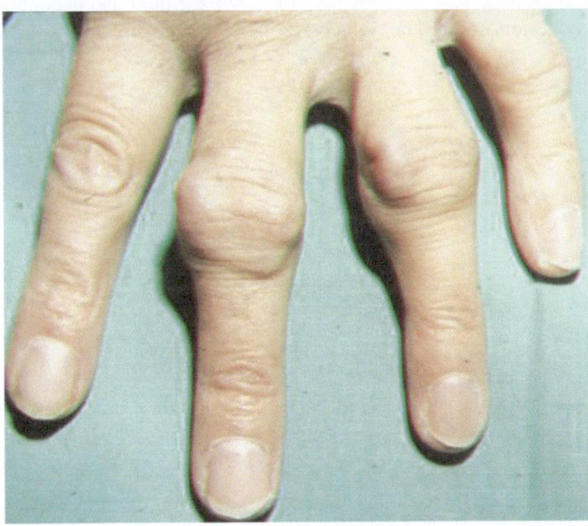

Fig. 5.4 Synovitis of PIP joint with synovial protrusion through the joint capsule and development of boutonniere deformity

References

1. Carl HD, Rech J. Large-joint synovectomy in the era of biological therapies. Z Rheumatol. 2011;70(1):9–13.
2. Klug S, Wittmann G, Weseloh G. Arthroscopic synovectomy of the knee joint in early cases of rheumatoid arthritis: follow-up results of a multicenter study. Arthroscopy. 2000;16(3):262–7.
3. Jüsten HP, Pommer S, Leeb I, Pilhofer C, Kisslinger E, Wessinghage D. Long-term results of open knee synovectomy in later cases of rheumatoid arthritis. Z Rheumatol. 1999;58(4):201–6.
4. Chalmers PN, Sherman SL, Raphael BS, Su EP. Rheumatoid synovectomy: does the surgical approach matter? Clin Orthop Relat Res. 2011;469(7):2062–71.
5. Goetz M, Klug S, Gelse K, Swoboda B, Carl HD. Combined arthroscopic and radiation synovectomy of the knee joint in rheumatoid arthritis: 14-year follow-up. Arthroscopy. 2011;27(1):52–9.
6. Carl HD, Schraml A, Swoboda B, Hohenberger G. Synovectomy of the hip in patients with juvenile rheumatoid arthritis. J Bone Joint Surg Am. 2007;89(9):1986–92.
7. Anders S, Schaumburger J, Kerl S, Schill S, Grifka J. Long-term results of synovectomy in the rheumatoid ankle joint. Z Rheumatol. 2007;66(7):595–602.
8. Kiekenbeck A, Preis M, Salzmann G. Rheumatoid shoulder: does minimally invasive therapy make sense? Z Rheumatol. 2008;67(6):462–70.
9. Smith AM, Sperling JW, O'Driscoll SW, Cofield RH. Arthroscopic shoulder synovectomy in patients with rheumatoid arthritis. Arthroscopy. 2006;22(1):50–6.
10. Tanaka N, Sakahashi H, Hirose K, Ishima T, Ishii S. Arthroscopic and open synovectomy of the elbow in rheumatoid arthritis. J Bone Joint Surg Am. 2006;88(3):521–5.
11. Kang HJ, Park MJ, Ahn JH, Lee SH. Arthroscopic synovectomy for the rheumatoid elbow. Arthroscopy. 2010;26(9):1195–202.
12. Dinges H, Fürst M, Rüther H, Schill S. Operative differential therapy of rheumatic wrists. Z Rheumatol. 2007;66(5):388–94.
13. Kim SJ, Jung KA. Arthroscopic synovectomy in rheumatoid arthritis of wrist. Clin Med Res. 2007;5(4):244–50.
14. Wei N, Delauter SK, Erlichman MS, Rozmaryn LM, Beard SJ, Henry DL. Arthroscopic synovectomy of the metacarpophalangeal joint in refractory rheumatoid arthritis: a technique. Arthroscopy. 1999;15(3):265–8.
15. Sekiya I, Kobayashi M, Taneda Y, Matsui N. Arthroscopy of the proximal interphalangeal and metacarpophalangeal joints in rheumatoid arthritis. Arthroscopy. 2002;18(3):292–7.
16. Kuzmanova SI, Atanassov AN, Andreev SA, Solakov PT. Minor and major complications of arthroscopic synovectomy of the knee joint performed by rheumatologist. Folia Med (Plovdiv). 2003;45(3):55–9.

Part II

Radiosynoviorthesis – Possible Side Effects and Complications

Radiosynovectomy: Introduction and Overview of the Literature

6

Ewald Kresnik

Contents

6.1 Introduction

Rheumatoid arthritis (RA) and local degenerative changes such as osteoarthritis (OA) are the most common reasons for synovitis that lead to chronic pain, swelling, destruction and dysfunction of the joints.

Systemic treatment including non-steroidal anti-inflammatory drugs (NSAIDs) as well as disease- modifying antirheumatic drugs (DMARDs), like biologicals, glucocorticoids (GC) and intraarticular GC injections is performed to control synovitis. In case with persisting synovitis, further therapy options are necessary.

E. Kresnik
Department of Nuclear Medicine, Private Hospital,
Dr. Walter Hochsteiner Strasse 4, Villach 9504, Austria
e-mail: kresnik@utanet.at

© Springer International Publishing Switzerland 2015
W.U. Kampen, M. Fischer (eds.), *Local Treatment of Inflammatory Joint Diseases: Benefits and Risks*, DOI 10.1007/978-3-319-16949-1_6

Studies have reported that surgical removal of the inflamed synovium can improve symptoms and function of the affected joints. However, due to insufficient removal of the inflamed synovial membrane in arthroscopic synovectomy, recurrence rate of synovitis was high [1–3].

Radiosynovectomy, also known as radiosynoviorthesis or RSO, is an important alternative to surgical or chemical synovectomy for the treatment of rheumatoid arthritis. The use of this therapy method had increased in the last years and is currently performed in about 100,000 joints per year in Europe.

A wide list of indications for RSO is reported in the literature, but the clinical outcome differs and depends on the primary disease, the type of the affected joint and the pre-existing degenerative changes.

6.2　Indications for Radiosynovectomy (RSO)

The indication for RSO is worked out in cooperation with the rheumatologists, orthopaedists and the nuclear medicine specialists. Only an expert in nuclear medicine is permitted to perform radiosynovectomy and is also responsible for the therapy.

RSO is reasonable if inflammation of the synovial membrane (synovitis) occurs. Therefore, before therapy diagnostic requirements such as arthrosonography and multiphase bone scintigraphy of the joints are mandatory to demonstrate synovitis (Fig. 6.1).

The main indications for RSO according to the European procedure guidelines for radiosynovectomy and with modifications to the German and Austrian

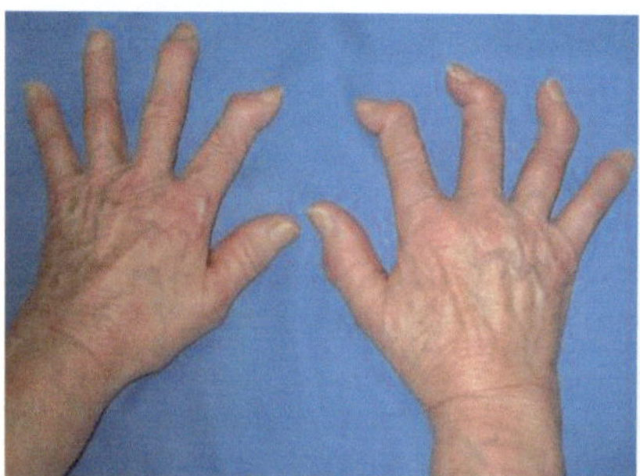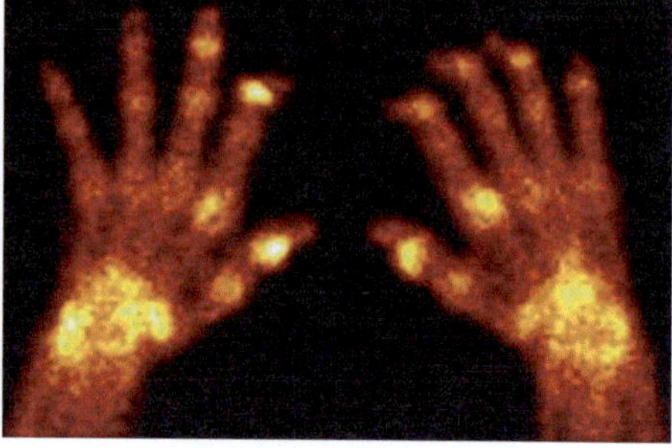

Fig. 6.1 A female patient, 72 years with rheumatoid arthritis of the hands. Before radiosynovectomy, scintigraphy is performed to clearly localize the inflamed joints. Tc-99m methylene diphosphonate (Tc-99m MDP) bone scintigraphy shows a typical symmetrical increased tracer uptake in both wrists and small finger joints due to synovitis (*right image*). Also in the distal interphalangeal joints, synovitis can be seen. The localization is not typical for rheumatoid arthritis and is secondary caused by degenerative changes

guidelines [4–6] are persisting synovitis after a 4- to 6-month systemic treatment in:

- Rheumatoid Arthritis
- Seronegative spondyloarthropathy (e.g. reactive or psoriatic arthritis)
- Other inflammatory joint diseases, e.g. Lyme disease and Behcet's disease
- Undifferentiated arthritis (where the arthritis is characterized by synovitis, synovial thickening or effusion)
- Persistent synovial effusion (e.g. after arthroscopic synovectomy)
- Persistent effusion after joint prosthesis
- Osteoarthritis (activated osteoarthrosis)
- Pigmented villonodular synovitis (PVNS)
- Haemophilic arthritis
- Contraindications
- Pregnancy
- Breast-feeding
- Local skin infection
- Acute rupture of popliteal cyst (Baker's cyst of the knee)
- Relative Contraindications
- The radiopharmaceuticals should only be used in children and young patients (<20 years), if the benefit of treatment is likely to outweigh the potential hazards.
- Extensive joint instability with bone destruction

6.3 Radiopharmaceuticals

The radionuclides that are injected into the articular cavity are phagocytized by the synovial cells. The irradiation leads to fibrotic and sclerosing changes of the synovial membrane and to an occlusion of the superficial capillaries. The inflammation as well as the proliferative and destructive process is stopped. Clinically, the pain and effusion of the treated joints, as well as the mobility get improved [7, 8].

In RSO β-emitting radionuclides are used.

Essential for the choice of the nuclides is the penetration depth of the emitted irradiation in correspondence to the thickness of the synovium and the nuclide's half-life. The most often used and approved nuclides for RSO in Europe are:

(Nuclide, half-life, mean/maximum penetration depth in tissue)
- Yttrium-90 citrate (Y-90, 2.7 days, 3.6/11 mm) – used for large joints like the knee joints

- Rhenium-186 sulphide (Re-186, 3.7 days, 1.2/3.7 mm) – used for medium-sized joints such as shoulder, elbow, wrist, hip and ankle
- Erbium-169 citrate (Er-169, 9.4 days, 0.3/1.0 mm) – used for small joints in the fingers and the toes, sterno- and acromioclavicular and temporomandibular

Furthermore, not so widespread used radionuclides for RSO are dysprosium-165 ferric hydroxide, holmium-166 hydroxyapatite and samarium-153 hydroxyapatite [9].

6.4 Radiosynovectomy in Rheumatoid Arthritis (RA)

The effectiveness of radiation synovectomy in rheumatoid arthritis was investigated by several authors.

In a meta- analysis 2,190 treated joints were evaluated [10]. There were 1,880 joints with rheumatoid arthritis and 37 patients with seronegative arthritis including psoriatic arthritis, ankylosing spondylitis and Reiter's disease. One hundred twenty-one had osteoarthritis. The period of observation was 1 year. The mean improvement rate for rheumatoid arthritis was 66.7 ± 15.4 %. For osteoarthritis the success rate was 56 ± 11 %. The results were dependent on the pre-existing morphological changes according to the American Association's staging criteria (Steinbrocker). The best results were achieved in patients without morphological changes. However, RSO in patients with changes according to Steinbrocker I was successful in 72.8 ± 12.3 % and in 64 ± 17.3 % in Steinbrocker II. Even in joints staged with Steinbrocker III and IV had a success rate of 52.4 ± 23.6 %.

Based on the clinical outcome after RSO, three groups were defined where RSO was indicated. In case of deformed or unstable joints, there was no clinical response. Therefore, RSO was not indicated (Table 6.1).

Most of the treated joints were large joints like knees (64 %). Medium-sized joints like shoulder, elbow, wrist, ankle and small finger joints were presented in 17 and 19 %.

Several studies were performed to determine the clinical response in the different types of joints.

6.4.1 Radiosynovectomy of Large Joints

Kampen et al. [11] reported in a summary of prospective studies in which 796 knee joints were treated using yttrium-90 colloid (Y-90) that the success rate ranged from 50 to 100 %. The overall follow-up duration was 6–36 months.

Several authors also compared yttrium-90 colloid (Y-90) with the intraarticular injection of corticosteroids. It turned out that RSO was effective in 78 and 70 % of RA patients in whom corticosteroids were ineffective [12, 13].

Furthermore, in a double-blind study by Urbanova et al. [14], the authors compared Y-90 in combination with corticosteroids. Corticosteroids alone and the

Table 6.1 Groups for RSO [10]

Group	Clinical response rate	Disease	Pre-existing morphological changes
A (appropriate)	>80 %	Rheumatoid arthritis Haemarthrosis in haemophilia Haemarthrosis in Willebrand's disease Villonodular synovitis	No changes
B (acceptable)	60–80 %	Rheumatoid arthritis Seronegative arthritis Osteoarthritis Repeating injection in previous responder	Steinbrocker I, II[a] Minimal or moderate
C (helpful)	<60 %	Rheumatoid arthritis Osteoarthritis	Steinbrocker III, IV[a] Severe destruction
D (not indicated)	No response	Need for surgical interventions Previous nonresponder Deformed joints Unstable joints	

[a]Classification according to the American Association's staging criteria (Steinbrocker)

combination with Y-90 colloid showed comparable efficacy in reduction of pain and effusion for a short time. But in the long term (after 12 months), Y-90 colloid was superior. The improvement was seen with the variables of pain, functional disability, joint tenderness and swelling.

Similar results were also found in a 6-year follow-up study by Grant et al. [15] in 21 patients with RA. After 6 years, 75 % of the patients that were treated initially with glucocorticoid (GC) needed other treatments (e.g. surgical synovectomy, knee arthroplasty, Y-90 reinjection) versus 66 % of patients in the RSO group ($p > 0.05$).

In another study [16] the combination therapy was also investigated in 15 patients with chronic pyrophosphate arthropathy of the knee. They found that all outcome parameters were significantly better for the combination of Y-90 and GC injection with regard to pain, stiffness, effusion, range of movement ($p < 0.01$) and joint circumference ($p < 0.05$). Therefore, the combination therapy was favoured in chronic pyrophosphate arthropathy.

It seems that the combination therapy is also the preferred therapy concept in clinical routine because, in a survey of radiation synovectomy in Europe, 60 % of the responders reported that they used corticosteroid co-injection with radiopharmaceuticals. Rheumatoid arthritis was the most prevalent disease in patients treated.

Regarding steroids, triamcinolone hexacetonide was most frequently used due of its relatively long residence time in joints.

It was also suggested that corticosteroids reduces lymph node uptake of radiocolloids [17, 18].

6.4.2 Surgical Synovectomy and Radiosynovectomy

Surgical synovectomy is well established in the local treatment of RA.

However, due to traumatization and insufficient removal of all pathological tissue with minimal arthroscopic synovectomy, the recurrence rate was high and amounted to 30 % in a long-term follow-up [2, 3].

Therefore, several authors reported the usefulness of the combination of arthroscopic subtotal synovectomy and radiosynovectomy.

In a recent study by Akmese et al. [19], the authors compared the combined arthroscopic synovectomy and RSO in the treatment of chronic non-specific synovitis of the knee. They found that the limitation of motion and effusion was significantly regressed. Also pain and synovial membrane thickness were significantly reduced (82 and 54 %). Clinically and radiologically on MRI, there was no recurrence after 3 years.

Similar results were also found from other authors. Kerschbaumer et al. [20] reported about significantly better long-term clinical results (8 years) in 141 knee joints that were treated with the combination therapy than patients that were treated with RSO alone.

Furthermore, in another study by Goetz et al. [21], 32 patients with RA of the knees were successfully treated with the combination therapy and also did not need any surgical re-intervention in 84, 44 and 34 % after 5, 10 and 14 years. Similar results were also found from other authors with better results for the combination therapy in the early stages of rheumatically swollen joints. Therefore, the authors suggested to perform the combined therapy for the treatment of early rheumatoid stages of the ankle joint. Additionally, open synovectomy should be preferred to arthroscopic synovectomy if tenosynovectomy is simultaneously required [22, 23].

Regarding the time of RSO, it was suggested to perform RSO 6 weeks after surgery, because after this time the postoperative edema had diminished and the surgical wound is almost closed to avoid any leakage of the injected radionuclide. Moreover, the postoperative inflammatory changes were at the maximum at this time and the efficacy of the anti-inflammatory effect of the RSO was thus increased [19].

Further studies are needed to establish this favourable therapy concept for the chronic non- specific synovitis in the long-term follow-up.

6.4.3 Radiosynovectomy in Knee Endoprosthesis

Radiosynovectomy was also under investigation for treating recurrent joint effusions after knee endoprosthesis.

First results about the usefulness of RSO in knee endoprosthesis were reported by Mödder et al. [24]. In their study 107 patients with chronic joint effusion due to "polyethylene disease" were treated with Y-90. In 93/107 (87 %) patients, joint effusion completely diminished after therapy.

In a recent study by Mayer-Wagner et al. [25], 55 patients with chronic joint effusion after endoprosthetic knee replacement were treated with Y-90 colloid.

Significant improvement in pain, effusion and function was seen in 54 %. Most of the patients in whom RSO treatment failed, complications like infection, loosening, allergy and trauma were detected.

In summary, RSO represents a valid therapeutic option in persistent effusion after joint prosthesis. However, in case of treatment failure, endoprosthetic complications should be excluded.

6.4.4 Radiosynovectomy of Medium- and Small-Sized Joints

Rhenium-186 is used for the hip, shoulder, elbow, wrist, ankle and subtalar joint and erbium-169 for finger and toe joints, acromio-/sternoclavicular joints and temporomandibular joints.

It was reported that the efficacy of RSO for medium-sized joints in RA varies from 60 to 90 % (Fig. 6.2a, b).

In two prospective studies by Göbel et al. [26, 27], the authors evaluated the efficacy of rhenium-186 for medium-sized joints ($n=50$) and erbium-169 for digital joints ($n=131$) in patients with RA. The injection of rhenium-186 and erbium-169 was combined with triamcinolonhexacetonid. The synovitis in the control groups was treated by the injection of cortisone alone. Follow-up time was 3 years. Pain, synovial swelling, joint motion and stage of radiological destruction (based on the staging by Larsen-Dale-Eek) were assessed.

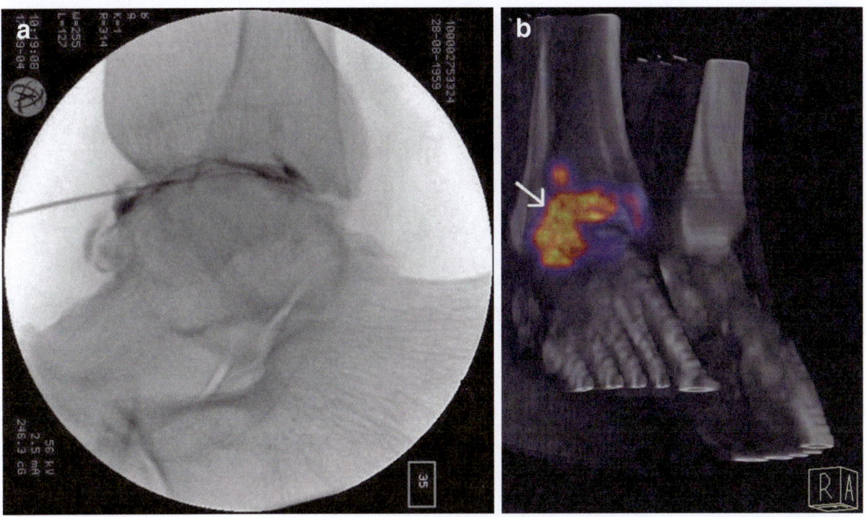

Fig. 6.2 (**a**) Arthrogram of the ankle joint during the RSO. The puncture needle can be seen on the left side. (**b**) Patient with rheumatoid arthritis was submitted for RSO of the right ankle joint. After the injection of 74 MBq rhenium-186, single-photon emission computed tomography (SPECT) is showing the distribution within the ankle joint (*arrow*)

Significantly better clinical results were achieved in the group with combined injection of radionuclide and cortisone. The results of the small metacarpophalangeal joints (MCP) and the medium-sized joints were comparably good. However, proximal interphalangeal joints (PIP) responded less than other joints, which was explained by a leakage of the nuclide due to increased movement during manual activities.

Therefore, a sufficient immobilization (up to 72 h) by using a finger splint is recommended to avoid leakage. However, according to the guidelines, if immobilization of the treated joint cannot be ensured, hospitalization is mandatory.

In the study mentioned above, the progression in radiological joint destruction correlated also with the clinical results and was significantly lower in comparison with the groups that were injected with cortisone alone.

The results are in concordance with other authors. In an international multicenter double-blind and placebo-controlled study on patients suffering from rheumatoid arthritis, 82 finger joints were investigated. After 6 months the results showed that pain and swelling significantly decreased (95 % vs. 42 %) and mobility increased (64 % vs. 42 %) after RSO [28].

In a similar study by van der Zant et al. [29], joints of the upper extremities were treated. The clinical effect was better when radionuclide plus cortisone was injected into the joints (69 %) than cortisone alone (29 %). Furthermore, there was no significant difference in clinical outcome for patients with RA and with non-RA. It seems that the destruction process of the joints as well as the localization also has an influence on the clinical effect of joint motion and pain.

In a study by Kraft et al. [30], the authors found that pain was significantly decreased after RSO, whereas the influence of joint motion was minimal. This was most likely due to the progressive destructive processes of the joints. Furthermore, the best results were observed for shoulders and elbows. Ankle joints responded worst.

Also other authors reported that the effect of RSO was higher for upper extremity than for lower extremity joints. It was supposed that this was due to mechanical forces in weight-bearing joints that could perpetuate the joint damage and recurrence of synovitis [12, 29, 31].

6.5   Radiosynovectomy in Osteoarthritis

Osteoarthritis (OA), which is also known as degenerative joint disease, is caused by mechanical abnormalities leading to a secondary synovitis with cartilage and subchondral bone destruction. Symptoms include joint pain, stiffness and sometimes joint effusion. Most often the weight-bearing joints of the lower extremities are affected. In finger polyarthrosis the distal interphalangeal (DIP) joints and/or proximal interphalangeal joints (PIP) and/or the first carpometacarpal (CMC) joints are involved.

RSO is indicated when synovitis occurs with pain and joint effusion.

In the literature the success rate ranges from 45 to 85 %. We also found in an own meta- analysis of 121 patients with OA that the mean success rate was 56 ± 11 %.

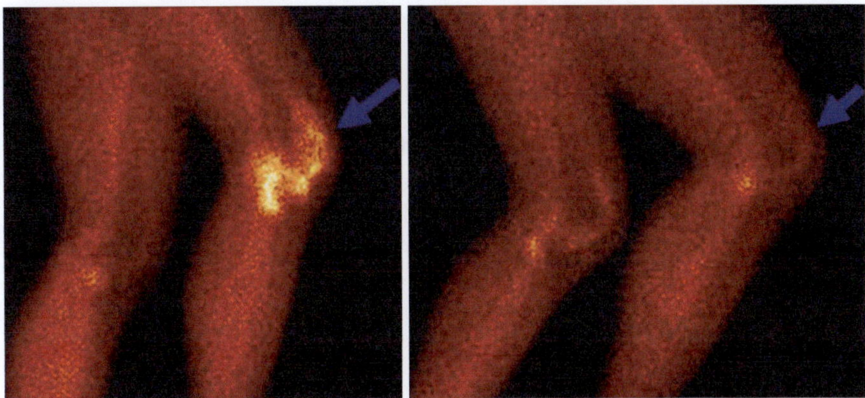

Fig. 6.3 A female patient, 50 years with chronic synovitis in osteoarthritis. Before radiosynovectomy, Tc-99m methylene diphosphonate (Tc-99m MDP) bone scintigraphy shows an increased tracer uptake in the early phase of scintigraphy of the right knee (*arrow* on the *left image*). Six months after radiosynovectomy, synovitis diminished and tracer uptake in Tc-99m MDP bone scintigraphy was significantly reduced (*arrow* on the *right image*)

The observation period was 1 year. Furthermore, it could be demonstrated that the improvement rate depended on pre-existing degenerative morphological changes. It turned out that the improvement rate was >80 % when there were no degenerative changes and 60–80 % in case of moderate changes (Fig. 6.3). However, the response rate decreased in cases of severe degenerative changes, but in clinical routine it was still classified as "helpful" with a success rate <60 % (Table 6.1).

Similar results were also found from other authors. It was reported that in patients with OA of the knee, the overall success rate in pain was 86 % and knee flexibility was improved in 65 %. Furthermore, the clinical improvement was inversely related to radiographic knee damage, patient's age and duration of the disease [32, 33].

Based on these results it seems that the therapy effect also depends on the underlying disease and the type of joint.

Zuderman et al. [34] reported that the success rate of RSO for the small-, medium- and large-sized joints were 89, 86 and 79 %. It was higher in RA (89 %) than in patients with OA (79 %). Furthermore, for the finger, ankle and wrist joints in RA, RSO was so promising that it should be preferred over the sole intraarticular corticoid injection.

Rau et al. [35] also found in a multicenter study that clinical outcome was significantly better in large joints for OA, but the response rate was similar for small- and large-sized joints in patients with RA.

However, in a study by Kampen et al. [36], the authors found that the therapy was also highly effective in digital joint OA with local synovitis. The best results were obtained in the thumb base joints. All patients also reported an improvement in their manual activities.

We also performed a double-blind controlled prospective study on 22 patients with local synovitis in OA of the thumb base joints. The effect of erbium-169 in combination with corticosteroids was compared to corticosteroid injection alone. The follow-up duration was 1 year.

It turned out that RSO in combination with steroids was significantly effective regarding reduction of pain, inflammation and improvement of the motion. Corticosteroids showed a significant reduction of pain for a limited time up to 6 weeks after injection, but after this time the pain worsened. There was also a disease progression in this group after 1 year [37].

6.6   Radiosynovectomy in Haemophilic Patients

Haemophilia is a hereditary disorder which causes bleeding into joints. Repeated joint bleedings cause joint and cartilage destruction. RSO is indicated when chronic synovitis occurs in chronic haemorrhagic arthropathy.

Several studies reported that the frequency of bleeding is reduced after RSO. Therefore, also the factor usage is reduced.

In an own meta-analysis of 15 patients with Willebrand's disease and 116 with haemophilia, a reduction of joint bleedings and factor usage after RSO was found in 91 ± 4.3 % [10].

This is in concordance with a recent study about haemophilic synovitis by Turkmen et al. [38]. The authors investigated 82 knee joints in a 10-year retrospective analysis. After 1, 3 and 5 years, there was no repeated bleeding in 89, 73 and 63 %, respectively. In addition, RSO was effective independent of the type of joint and the degree of synovial hypertrophy. However, it was also reported that the more severe synovites and the knee joints reqired more injections than the elbow or the ankle joints [39, 40].

Kastersen et al. [41] also reported a reduction of the frequency of joint bleeding after RSO in 94 % during the first year. Patients with minor or no radiological changes of the joints showed the best results. This is in concordance with other authors of more than 250 treated joints. Furthermore,RSO turned out to be safe and highly cost effective in comparison to surgical synovectomy and should be performed early before the appearance of articular cartilage damage [42–44].

> **Conclusion**
>
> Radiosynovectomy (RSO) represents an effective therapy method in the treatment regime of inflammatory joint diseases. Several indications for RSO according to the guidelines are reported in the literature.
>
> RSO is appropriate in the treatment of rheumatic arthritis and haemophilic arthropathy with a high clinical response rate. RSO also provides acceptable clinical results in patients with osteoarthritis according to the degenerative changes.
>
> Large- as well as medium- and small-sized joints are suitable for RSO.
>
> The co-injection of glucocorticoids and radiation synovectomy provide favourable clinical results and is therefore most often performed in clinical routine.

In case of arthroscopic synovectomy, the combination with RSO provides significantly better clinical results than the surgical method alone.

Therefore, close cooperation with the rheumatologists and orthopaedists is necessary to consider RSO in each patient to ensure optimal medical care.

References

1. Matsui N, Taneda Y, Ohta H, Itoh T, Tsuboguchi S. Arthroscopic versus open synovectomy in the rheumatoid knee. Int Orthop. 1989;13:17–20.
2. Roch – Bras F, Daures JP, Legouffe MC, Sany J, Combe B. Treatment of chronic knee synovitis with arthroscopic synovectomy: longterm results. J Rheumatol. 2002;6:1171–5.
3. Blahut J. Synovectomy of the knee joint. Acta Chir Orthop Traumatol Czech. 2003;70:371–6.
4. Clunie G, Fischer M. EANM procedure guidelines for radiosynovectomy. Eur J Nucl Med Mol Imaging. 2003;30:12–6.
5. Farahati J, Reiners C, Fischer M, Mödder G, Franke C, Mahlstedt J, Sörensen H. Guidelines for radiosynoviorthesis. Nuklearmedizin. 1999;38:254–5.
6. Kresnik E, Panholzer P, Pirich C, Gabriel M. Austrian Association of Nuclear Medicine Radiosynoviorthesis guideline. 2013. www.ogn.at.
7. Gratz S, Göbel D, Behr TM, Herrmann A, Becker W. Correlation between radiation dose, synovial thickness, and efficacy of radiosynoviorthesis. J Rheumatol. 1999;26:1242–9.
8. Myers SL, Slowman SD, Brandt KD. Radiation synovectomy stimulates glycosaminoglycan synthesis by normal articular cartilage. J Lab Clin Med. 1989;114:27–35.
9. Fischer M, Mödder G. Radionuclide therapy of inflammatory joint diseases. Nucl Med Commun. 2002;23:829–31.
10. Kresnik E, Mikosch P, Gallowitsch HJ, Jesenko R, Just H, Kogler D, Gasser J, Heinisch M, Unterweger O, Kumnig G, Gomez I, Lind P. Clinical outcome of radiosynoviorthesis: a meta-analysis including 2190 treated joints. Nucl Med Commun. 2002;23:683–8.
11. Kampen WU, Voth M, Pinkert J, Krause A. Therapeutic status of radiosynoviorthesis of the knee with yttrium [90Y] colloid in rheumatoid arthritis and related indications. Rheumatology. 2007;46:16–24.
12. Jahangier ZN, Moolenburgh JD, Jacobs JW, Serdijn H, Bijlsma JW. The effect of radiation synovectomy in patients with persistent arthritis: a prospective study. Clin Exp Rheumatol. 2001;19:417–24.
13. Menkes CJ. Controlled trial of intra-articular Yttrium-90 osmic acid and triamcinolone. San Francisco: XIV Int Congr Rheum; 1997.
14. Urabnova Z, Gatterova J, Olejarova M, Pavelka K. Radiosynoviorthesis with Y90- results of a clinical study. Ees Revmatol. 1997;5:140–2.
15. Grant AN, Bellamy N, Fryday-Field K, Disney T, Driedger A, Hobby Y. Double-blind randomized controlled trial and six-year open follow-up of yttrium-90 radiosynovectomy versus triamcinolone hexacetonide in persistent rheumatoid knee synovitis. Inflammopharmacol. 1992;1:231–8.
16. Doherty M, Dieppe PA. Effect of intra-articular yttrium-90 on chronic pyrophosphate arthropathy of the knee. Lancet. 1981;2:1243–6.
17. Derendorf H, Möllmann H, Grüner A, Haack D, Gyselby G. Pharmacokinetics and pharmacodynamics of glucocorticoid suspensions after intra-articular administration. Clin Pharmacol Ther. 1986;39:313–7.
18. Clunie G, Ell P. A survey of radiation synovectomy in Europe, 1991–1993. Eur J Nucl Med. 1995;22:970–6.
19. Akmeşe R, Yildiz KI, Işik Ç, Tecimel O, Bilgetekin YG, Firat A, Özakinci H, Bozkurt M. Combined arthroscopic synovectomy and radiosynoviorthesis in the treatment of chronic non-specific synovitis of the knee. Arch Orthop Trauma Surg. 2013;133:1567–73.

20. Kerschbaumer F, Kandziora F, Herresthal J, Hertel A, Hör G. Combined arthroscopic and radiation synovectomy in rheumatoid arthritis. Orthopade. 1998;27:188–96.
21. Goetz M, Klug S, Gelse K, Swoboda B, Carl HD. Combined arthroscopic and radiation synovectomy of the knee joint in rheumatoid arthritis: 14-year follow-up. Arthroscopy. 2011;27:52–9.
22. Rittmeister M, Böhme T, Rehart S, Kerschbaumer F. Treatment of the ankle joint in rheumatoid arthritis with surgical and radiation synovectomy. Orthopade. 1999;28:785–91.
23. Rehart S, Arnold I, Fürst M. Conservative local therapy of inflammation of joints: local invasive forms of therapy. Z Rheumatol. 2007;66:382–7.
24. Mödder G. Radiosynoviorthesis after total knee replacement: effective therapy of "polyethylene disease". Nuklearmedizin. 2001;24:97–103.
25. Mayer-Wagner S, Mutzel B, Mayer W, Fulghum C, Simon G, Linke R, Jansson V. Radiosynoviorthesis for treating recurrent joint effusions after endoprosthetic knee replacement. Clin Nucl Med. 2012;37:727–31.
26. Göbel D, Gratz S, von Rothkirch T, Becker W. Chronic polyarthritis and radiosynoviorthesis: a prospective, controlled study of injection therapy with erbium 169 and rhenium 186. Z Rheumatol. 1997;56:207–13.
27. Göbel D, Gratz S, von Rothkirch T, Becker W, Willert HG. Radiosynoviorthesis with rhenium-186 in rheumatoid arthritis: a prospective study of three treatment regimens. Rheumatol Int. 1997;17:105–8.
28. Kahan A, Mödder G, Menkes CJ, Verrier P, Devaux JY, Bonmartin A, De Rycke Y, Manil L, Chossat F, Tebib J. 169-Erbium-citrate synoviorthesis after failure of local corticosteroid injections to treat rheumatoid arthritis-affected finger joints. Clin Exp Rheumatol. 2004;22:722–6.
29. van der Zant FM, Jahangier ZN, Moolenburgh JD, Swen WA, Boer RO, Jacobs JW. Clinical effect of radiation synovectomy of the upper extremity joints: a randomised, double-blind, placebo-controlled study. Eur J Nucl Med Mol Imaging. 2007;34:212–8.
30. Kraft O, Kašparek R. Effectiveness of radiosynoviorthesis in the treatment of chronic synovitis of small and middle-sized joints affected by rheumatoid arthritis. Hell J Nucl Med. 2011;14:251–4.
31. van der Zant FM, Boer RO, Moolenburgh JD, Jahangier ZN, Bijlsma JW, Jacobs JW. Radiation synovectomy with (90)Yttrium, (186)Rhenium and (169)Erbium: a systematic literature review with meta-analyses. Clin Exp Rheumatol. 2009;27:130–9.
32. Markou P, Chatzopoulos D. Yttrium-90 silicate radiosynovectomy treatment of painful synovitis in knee osteoarthritis. Results after 6 months. Hell J Nucl Med. 2009;12:33–6.
33. Farahati J, Schulz G, Wendler J, Körber C, Geling M, Kenn W, Schmeider P, Reidemeister C, Reiners C. Multivariate analysis of factors influencing the effect of radiosynovectomy. Nuklearmedizin. 2002;41:114–9.
34. Zuderman L, Liepe K, Zöphel K, Andreeff M, Kotzerke J, Luboldt W. Radiosynoviorthesis (RSO): influencing factors and therapy monitoring. Ann Nucl Med. 2008;22:735–41.
35. Rau H, Lohmann K, Franke C, Goretzki G, Lemb MA, Müller J, Panholzer PJ, Stelling E, Spitz J. Multicenter study of radiosynoviorthesis. Clinical outcome in osteoarthritis and other disorders with concomitant synovitis in comparison with rheumatoid arthritis. Nuklearmedizin. 2004;43:57–62.
36. Kampen WU, Hellweg L, Massoudi-Nickel S, Czech N, Brenner W, Henze E. Clinical efficacy of radiation synovectomy in digital joint osteoarthritis. Eur J Nucl Med Mol Imaging. 2005;32:575–80.
37. Kresnik E, Igerc I, Gallowitsch HJ, Mikosch P, Maier U, Pfandlsteiner T, Lind P. Radiosynovectomy with erbium-169 in osteoarthritis of the thumb base joints: a double-blind controlled prospective study in comparison to corticosteroid injection. 2014: data in preparation for publication.
38. Turkmen C, Kilicoglu O, Dikici F, Bezgal F, Kuyumcu S, Gorgun O, Taser O, Zulfikar B. Survival analysis of Y-90 radiosynovectomy in the treatment of haemophilic synovitis of the knee: a 10-year retrospective review. Haemophilia. 2014;20:45–50.

39. Zulfikar B, Turkmen C, Kilicoglu O, Dikici F, Bezgal F, Gorgun O, Taser O. Long-term outcomes in haemophilic synovitis after radiosynovectomy using rhenium-186: a single-centre experience. Haemophilia. 2013;19:275–80.
40. Corte-Rodriguez H, Rodriguez-Merchan EC, Jimenez-Yuste V. What patient, joint and isotope characteristics influence the response to radiosynovectomy in patients with haemophilia? Haemophilia. 2011;17:990–8.
41. Kasteren ME, Nováková IR, Boerbooms AM, Lemmens JA. Long term follow up of radiosynovectomy with yttrium-90 silicate in haemophilic haemarthrosis. Ann Rheum Dis. 1993;52:548–50.
42. Brecelj J, Bole V, Benedik-Dolnicar M, Grmek M. The co effect of prophylaxis and radiosynovectomy on bleeding episodes in haemophilic synovitis. Haemophilia. 2008;14:513–7.
43. Rampersad AG, Shapiro AD, Rodriguez-Merchan EC, Maahs JA, Akins S, Jimenez-Yuste V. Radiosynovectomy: review of the literature and report from two haemophilia treatment centers. Blood Coagul Fibrinolysis. 2013;24:465–70.
44. Rodriguez- Merchan EC. Cartilage damage in the haemophilic joints: pathophysiology, diagnosis and management. Blood Coagul Fibrinolysis. 2012;23:179–83.

Dosimetry and Radiation Exposure of Patients

7

Michael Lassmann

Contents

7.1 Introduction

Radiosynoviorthesis is a local radionuclide therapy of inflamed synovial membranes involving either Y-90, Er-169, or Re-186. Although the radioactive substance is not supposed to leave the joint after the injection, it might leak to the adjacent lymph nodes and, subsequently, to the remainder of the body. Data on this leakage to regional lymph nodes is provided in various publications [1–5]. Furthermore, since faint uptake in the liver can be seen in some patients, it can be assumed that a fraction of the radioactively labeled colloids reach the blood circulation and are taken up by the reticuloendothelial system.

M. Lassmann
Klinik und Poliklinik für Nuklearmedizin, Universitätsklinikum Würzburg,
Oberdürrbacher Str. 6, Würzburg D – 97080, Germany
e-mail: lassmann_m@ukw.de

© Springer International Publishing Switzerland 2015
W.U. Kampen, M. Fischer (eds.), *Local Treatment of Inflammatory Joint Diseases: Benefits and Risks*, DOI 10.1007/978-3-319-16949-1_7

The purpose of this chapter is to provide an assessment of leakage rates, absorbed and effective doses to the remainder of the body by leakage, by external irradiation from the joint itself, and absorbed doses to the neighboring lymph nodes.

Due to the low amount of activity injected and the physical properties of the radionuclides used, the exposure of relatives and the public by these patients is extremely low and can be neglected.

7.2 Leakage Rate After Injection

One of the major sources for radiation exposure of the patient is leakage of the radioactive compound from the joint to the adjacent lymph nodes or other organs and tissues. A number of authors reported data on leakage rates.

Gedik et al. [5] determined the leakage rate 48 h after administration of Y-90 or Re-186 in 35 patients with persisting synovitis. The mean leakage of 19 joints treated with Y-90-citrate was 3.2 % (maximum 13 %) and of 21 joints treated with Y-90-silicate 2.3 % (maximum 5 %). There was no statistically significant difference. In addition Gedik et al. [5] observed a mean leakage in 13 patients treated with Re-186-sulfide of 2.5 % (maximum 6 %). Turkmen et al. [6] published leakage data showing that the 50 % percentile of the leakage was 1.8 % and the 84.1 % percentile was 4.8 %. Turkmen et al. [7] determined leakage rates in 20 juvenile hemophilia patients by measuring the uptake with a gamma camera 48 h after injection. The authors observed, in 11 patients, a mean leakage of 0.2 % in lymph nodes and 4.7 % in the liver (maximum, 7.6 %).

Klett et al. [8] measured, for ten patients, the leakage 3 days after injection of 50–60 MBq Re-186. Eight of the ten patients showed a mean leakage of 3.9 % (maximum, 23.4 %) to the axillary lymph nodes. Two patients showed uptake in the liver, one in the spleen.

Van der Zant et al. [4] reported on leakage of Er-169 and Re-186 in 31 patients with arthritis by bremsstrahlung scintigraphy. The mean leakage was 2.1 % for lymph nodes (Re-186, maximum 9.9 %), 0.11 % (Er-169, 1 case), and for liver/spleen 0.5 % (maximum 6.8 %). Van der Zant et al. [9] also determined the leakage from the ankles about 24 h after the injection of 75 MBq Re-186 by imaging. The mean leakage to lymph nodes (2.4 ± 3 %) was higher than to the liver (0.8 ± 1.7 %).

Manil et al. determined the leakage rate from scintigraphic images with the isotope Re-186 using a dual-head gamma camera [3]. Whole body and static images of the injection sites and lymph node chains were obtained. A measurable extra-articular activity was only found in drainage lymph nodes and in the hepatosplenic area. The proportion of the whole body activity in lymph nodes was 4.5 % at 6 h, 4.4 % at 24 h, and 6.0 % at day 7. For the hepatosplenic area, the corresponding results were 0.9 % at 6 h, 1.1 % at 24 h, and 2.1 % at day 7. Van der Zant et al. [9] observed the leakage from the ankles about 24 h after the injection of 75 MBq by Re-186 by imaging. The mean leakage to lymph nodes (2.4 ± 3 %) was higher than to the liver (0.8 ± 1.7 %). The maximal observed leakage to a single lymph node was 4 % and to the liver 5.5 %. For 12 patients with hemophilia, Grmek et al. [2]

calculated leakage rates after the injection of Re-186 colloids. The author observed a mean leakage of 20 ± 10 % (maximum, 40 %). Four of the 12 patients showed uptake in lymph nodes. Overall, leakage rates up to 8 % have been observed.

7.3   Radiation Exposure of Healthy Organs

7.3.1   Generic Model

For calculating the absorbed doses, data on distribution of colloids were taken from the ICRP Publication 53 [10]. In this publication, slightly different data sets are provided for large colloids (diameter 100–1,000 nm) and for small colloids (diameter <100 nm) for the conditions "normal liver."

As suggested in the ICRP Publication 53, immediate uptake by the listed tissues is assumed. Furthermore, it is assumed that the biological half-life in the specified tissues is long compared with the physical half-life of the radionuclide. Under the above assumptions, the residence time in an organ is determined by the physical half-life, the organ uptake, and the percentage of injected activity that leaks out of the joint:

$$\text{Residence time per \% of leakage} = \text{Organ uptake} \times \text{physical half life} / \ln(2) / 100$$

With a half-life of the physical decay of Y-90, Er-169, and Re-186, the resulting residence times per % of leakage were calculated. With these residence times, the absorbed doses to healthy organs and tissues were calculated using software OLINDA/EXM [11]. Organ doses and effective doses as a function of the percentage of leakage are displayed in Table 7.1 for the isotopes under consideration.

7.3.2   Observed Absorbed Doses

According to data on Y-90 published by Klett et al. [12], the median absorbed doses to the liver and spleen were 62 and 62 mGy, respectively. Somewhat higher mean doses for the liver, spleen, and kidneys (265, 119, and 671 mGy) were reported by Gratz et al. [1]. The organ doses to the liver and spleen published by Klett et al. [12] are consistent with mean leakage to the blood system of about 2 %. While the spleen doses reported by Gratz et al. [1] are consistent with 2 % leakage, the liver doses are higher requiring 8 % leakage. The high kidney doses are not consistent with the model assumptions.

Reliable measurements of the whole body activity after administration of Er-169 are not available as almost no direct radiation leaves the body. Manil et al. [3] measured the total blood activity after Er-169 therapy of finger joints in 11 patients and found less than 1 % of the administered activity in all but 1 patient with scintigraphic evidence of extra-articular injection. The effective dose was maximal for this patient and was estimated to be 0.045 mSv/MBq. For Er-169 Gratz et al. [1] estimated the radiation dose to the whole body to be 0.11 mGy/MBq.

Table 7.1 Radiation dose for the reference adult for colloids per % of leakage

Target organ	Y-90 labeled colloids		Er-169 labeled colloids		Re-186 labeled colloids	
	Large colloids (>100 nm) mGy/MBq/ %leakage	Small colloids (<100 nm) mGy/MBq/ %leakage	Large colloids (>100 nm) mGy/MBq/ %leakage	Large colloids (>100 nm) mGy/MBq/ %leakage	Large colloids (>100 nm) mGy/MBq/ %leakage	Small colloids (<100 nm) mGy/MBq/ %leakage
Kidneys	6.76E-04	3.38E-04	2.61E-04	1.31E-04	5.82E-04	4.13E-04
Liver	1.83E-01	1.83E-01	7.05E-02	7.02E-02	9.25E-02	9.25E-02
Ovaries	6.76E-04	3.38E-04	2.61E-04	1.31E-04	3.88E-04	2.19E-04
Red marrow	2.00E-02	2.95E-02	1.06E-02	1.56E-02	1.08E-02	1.59E-02
Osteogenic cells	1.34E-02	1.91E-02	5.47E-03	7.17E-03	7.08E-03	9.86E-03
Spleen	2.64E-01	2.64E-01	1.05E-01	1.05E-01	1.37E-01	1.37E-01
Testes	6.76E-04	3.38E-04	2.61E-04	1.31E-04	3.50E-04	1.76E-04
Uterus	6.76E-04	3.38E-04	2.61E-04	1.31E-04	3.79E-04	2.08E-04
Other organs	6.76E-04	3.38E-04	2.61E-04	1.31E-04	<1E-03	<1E-03
Total body	6.76E-03	6.76E-03	2.61E-03	2.61E-03	3.49E-03	3.48E-03
	mSv/MBq/ % leakage	*mSv/MBq/ % leakage*	*mSv/MBq/ % leakage*	*mSv/MBq/ % leakage*	*mSv/MBq/ % leakage*	*mSv/MBq/ % leakage*
Effective dose	1.88E-02	1.97E-02	7.67E-03	8.20E-03	9.72E-03	1.02E-02

For Re-186 the effective dose, according to Manil et al. [3], calculated from the whole body dose due to gamma emission from injection point(s) and uptake foci, as well as from organ doses due to blood activity, was 380 µSv/MBq. According to Manil et al. [3], the radiation dose to the blood ranged between 0.07 and 0.88 mGy/MBq (mean value: 0.34 mGy/MBq). Gratz et al. [1] determined the doses to the hands and other organs by gamma imaging. The authors evaluated whole body and organ time-activity curves using conjugate views to generate residence times. In the 23 cases injected with 74 MBq Re-186 for the ankles ($n=7$), elbows ($n=3$), and wrists ($n=4$) and 111 MBq for shoulders ($n=8$) and hips ($n=1$)], the mean absorbed doses to the whole body, liver, spleen, and kidneys were 53 ± 27 mGy, 100 ± 81 mGy, 203 ± 228 mGy, and 94 ± 113 mGy, respectively. Van der Zant et al. [9] observed an absorbed dose to the liver of 7.5 mGy. Manil et al. [3] and van der Zant et al. [9] have published data of Re-186 uptakes in the hepatosplenic area which are consistent with leakage to the blood system of about 1–2 %. The corresponding values for the mean whole body dose and the organ doses published by Gratz et al. [1] are much higher requiring 50 % leakage or even more.

7.4   Radiation Dose from Penetrating Radiation from the Joint

The mean synovial thickness in joints treated with Y-90 is 6.8 mm [1]. The energy loss of the beta radiation ($E_{max}=2.27$ MeV, range 10 mm in water) is expected to be mainly in the synovia and the production of bremsstrahlung will be similar to that in water. An experimentally verified calculation of the radiation dose from bremsstrahlung of Y-90 has been published by Stabin et al. [13]. Production of bremsstrahlung is proportional to the square of the beta energy. The doses in 5, 10, 20, and 30 cm distance are 0.056, 0.011, 0.0015, and 0.0004 mGy/MBq, respectively.

The dose to organs and gonads from the bremsstrahlung from 200 MBq Y-90 in the knee is less than 0.1 mSv. The gonad dose per % of leakage into the inguinal lymph nodes can be estimated to be less than 0.1 mSv for males and approximately 0.02 mSv for females. The dose from bremsstrahlung from the inguinal lymph nodes to other organs is negligible.

The γ-dose rate constant for the penetrating radiation of Re-186 is 2.4 µSv $\times$ m^2/h/GBq. With an attenuation coefficient (energy absorption coefficient) of 0.03/cm the doses in 10, 15, and 30 cm distance are calculated to 0.023, 0.009, and 0.001 mGy/MBq, respectively. The expected radiation dose to the gonads (mean distance 10–15 cm) from a therapy of a hip with 150 MBq Re-186 is between 1.4 and 3.5 mSv. The gonad dose from therapies of other joints with less activity will not exceed 0.1 mSv.

The mean synovial thickness in joints treated with Er-169 is 2.4 mm [1]. The beta radiation ($E_{max}=0.35$ MeV, range 1 mm in water) is expected to be stopped in the synovia and the production of bremsstrahlung will be similar to that in water. Production of bremsstrahlung is proportional to the square of the beta energy. Taking into account the square of the ratio of the mean beta energies and differences in emission probabilities (EP) and residence times (RT) and neglecting differences in the energy absorption coefficient which are expected to be small, the dose per MBq administered is expected to be

$$D_{\text{Er-169}} = D_{\text{Y-90}} \times \left(E_{\text{Er-169}} / E_{\text{Y-90}} \right)^2 \times \text{RT}_{\text{Er-169}} / \text{RT}_{\text{Y-90}} \times \text{EP}_{\text{Er-169}} / \text{EP}_{\text{Y-90}} = 0.04 \times D_{\text{Y-90}}$$

With $D_{\text{Y-90}}$ taken from [13], the dose from Er-169 bremsstrahlung in 10 cm distance is 4×10^{-4} mGy/MBq and, therefore, negligible.

The mean synovial thickness in joints treated with Re-186 is 3.7 mm [1]. The beta radiation ($E_{\text{max}} = 1.05$ MeV, range 4 mm in water) is expected to be stopped in the synovia and the production of bremsstrahlung will be similar to that in water. Taking into account the square of the ratio of the mean beta energies and differences in emission probabilities (EP) and residence times (RT) and neglecting differences in the energy absorption coefficient which are expected to be small, the dose per MBq administered is expected to be

$$D_{\text{Re-186}} = D_{\text{Y-90}} \times \left(E_{\text{Re-186}} / E_{\text{Y-90}} \right)^2 \times \text{RT}_{\text{Re-186}} / \text{RT}_{\text{Y-90}} \times \text{EP}_{\text{Re-186}} / \text{EP}_{\text{Y-90}} = 0.2 \times D_{\text{Y-90}}$$

With $D_{\text{Y-90}}$ taken from Stabin et al. [13], the absorbed doses from bremsstrahlung from Re-186 in 10, 15, and 30 cm distance are 0.002, 0.0006, and 0.0001 mGy/MBq, respectively. The absorbed dose from the bremsstrahlung is an order of magnitude below the dose from the γ-radiation, and the corresponding absorbed dose to the gonads from a therapy of a hip with 150 MBq Re-186 is less than 0.3 mSv.

7.5 Radiation Exposure of the Lymph Nodes

7.5.1 Generic Model

For Y-90 the dose to a spherical node with homogeneous activity concentration and a mass of 1 g is 380 mGy per MBq administered activity and per % of the residence time accounting for the node. The correspondent values for nodes with other masses are 2,610 mGy/MBq/% at 0.1 g, 702 mGy/MBq/% at 0.5 g, and 202 mGy/MBq/% at 2 g. Due to the high energy of the beta particles emitted by Y-90, an increasing fraction of the radiation energy is deposited outside the node for decreasing diameters, and the absorbed fraction is shape dependent. The values given above will overestimate the dose in nodes with pronounced nonspherical shapes. Using the same assumptions for the biokinetics as for Re-186, the doses to the affected lymph nodes are 366 mGy/MBq/% if the activity is distributed in a mass of 1 g, 183 mGy/MBq/% if the mass is 2 g, and 91 mGy/MBq/% if the total mass is 4 g.

For Er-169 the dose to a spherical node with homogeneous activity concentration is 190 mGy*g/MBq/%. The dose is dependent on the residence time in the lymph node masses and the total mass of the involved lymph nodes but is almost independent of size and shape of individual lymph nodes. Using the same assumptions for the biokinetics as for Re-186, the doses to the affected lymph nodes are

190 mGy/MBq/% if the activity is distributed in a mass of 1 g, 95 mGy/MBq/% if the mass is 2 g, and 48 mGy/MBq/% if the total mass is 4 g.

For Re-186, according to the sphere model in OLINDA/EXM [11], the dose to a spherical node with homogeneous activity concentration and a mass of 1 g is 234 mGy per MBq administered activity and per % of the residence time accounting for the node. The correspondent values for nodes with other masses are 2,150 mGy/MBq/% at 0.1 g, 458 mGy/MBq/% at 0.5 g, and 119 mGy/MBq/% at 2 g. The product of dose and mass is 225 mGy*g/MBq/% ±5 % for all sizes indicating that the dose is dependent on the residence time in the lymph node masses and on the total mass of the involved lymph nodes but is almost independent of size and shape of individual lymph nodes.

The time-activity function of the activity leaking out of the joint is undefined. Activity release may be limited to a short time interval after the administration; it may occur sporadically after joint movement, or activity may leak out of the joint continuously. With the simplified assumption of a short-term leakage immediately after activity administration and for the worst-case scenario that the activity taken up by the lymph node masses stays there until decay, the percentage of the residence time accounting to the lymph node mass is identical to the uptake in % of the administered activity. The doses to the affected lymph nodes are 225 mGy/MBq/% if the activity is distributed in a mass of 1 g, 113 mGy/MBq/% if the mass is 2 g, and 56 mGy/MBq/% if the total mass is 4 g.

7.5.2 Observed Absorbed Doses

For Er-169 Gratz et al. [1] observed an absorbed dose of 2.3 ± 2 Gy (62 mGy/MBq) for single lymph nodes, van der Zant et al. 3 Gy [4].

For Re-186 Gratz et al. [1] report doses to lymph node masses of 25.9 ± 53.8 Gy (maximum 189 Gy) and to single lymph nodes of 14.7 ± 11.2 (maximum 63 Gy) after the application of 74–111 MBq Re-186. Van der Zant et al. determined the maximal observed dose to a single lymph node to 35 Gy [9]. For 12 patients with hemophilia, Grmek et al. [2] calculated absorbed doses after the injection of Re-186 colloids. The author observed a mean absorbed dose in those lymph nodes of 15 Gy. Van der Zant et al. [11] calculated the doses using the MIRD algorithms and found a maximum absorbed dose of 86 Gy.

Data for Y-90 are not available.

Conclusions

For RSO the exposure to organs/tissues other than the treated joint is negligible if there is no leakage. If there is leakage, the absorbed dose to neighboring lymph nodes could be higher than a few hundred mGy, thus leaving the deterministic range of radiation effects however depending upon the amount of leakage and the size of the lymph node of the individual patient. For the remainder of the body, the highest exposure of much less than one Gray is expected in the liver. The external exposure by the joint itself is low and does not contribute significantly to the patient exposure.

References

1. Gratz S, Gobel D, Behr TM, Herrmann A, Becker W. Correlation between radiation dose, synovial thickness, and efficacy of radiosynoviorthesis. J Rheumatol. 1999;26(6):1242–9.
2. Grmek M, Milcinski M, Fettich J, Brecelj J. Radiation exposure of hemophiliacs after radiosynoviorthesis with [186]Re colloid. Cancer Biother Radiopharm. 2007;22(3):417–22. doi:10.1089/cbr.2006.322.
3. Manil L, Voisin P, Aubert B, Guerreau D, Verrier P, Lebegue L, Wargnies JP, Di Paola M, Barbier Y, Chossat F, Menkes CJ, Tebib J, Devaux JY, Kahan A. Physical and biological dosimetry in patients undergoing radiosynoviorthesis with erbium-169 and rhenium-186. Nucl Med Commun. 2001;22(4):405–16.
4. van der Zant FM, Jahangier ZN, Gommans GG, Moolenburgh JD, Jacobs JW. Radiation synovectomy of the upper extremity joints: does leakage from the joint to non-target organs impair its therapeutic effect? Appl Radiat Isot. 2007;65(6):649–55. doi:10.1016/j.apradiso.2007.01.010. S0969-8043(07)00030-9 [pii].
5. Gedik GK, Ugur O, Atilla B, Pekmezci M, Yildirim M, Seven B, Varoglu E. Comparison of extraarticular leakage values of radiopharmaceuticals used for radionuclide synovectomy. Ann Nucl Med. 2006;20(3):183–8.
6. Turkmen C, Ozturk S, Unal SN, Zulfikar B, Taser O, Sanli Y, Cefle K, Kilicoglu O, Palanduz S. The genotoxic effects in lymphocyte cultures of children treated with radiosynovectomy by using yttrium-90 citrate colloid. Cancer Biother Radiopharm. 2007;22(3):393–9. doi:10.1089/cbr.2006.328.
7. Turkmen C, Ozturk S, Unal SN, Zulfikar B, Taser O, Sanli Y, Cefle K, Kilicoglu O, Palanduz S, Ozel S. Monitoring the genotoxic effects of radiosynovectomy with Re-186 in paediatric age group undergoing therapy for haemophilic synovitis. Haemophilia. 2007;13(1):57–64. doi:10.1111/j.1365-2516.2006.01406.x.
8. Klett R, Puille M, Steiner D, Bauer R. Radiation synovectomy of the knee joint: evaluation of bremsstrahlung-detection by using a corpse phantom. Nuklearmedizin Nucl Med. 2006;45(1):57–61. doi:10.1267/NUKL06010057.
9. van der Zant FM, Jahangier ZN, Moolenburgh JD, van der Zee W, Boer RO, Jacobs JW. Radiation synovectomy of the ankle with 75 MBq colloidal [186]rhenium-sulfide: effect, leakage, and radiation considerations. J Rheumatol. 2004;31(5):896–901. 0315162X-31-896 [pii].
10. ICRP. Publication 53: radiation dose to patients from radiopharmaceuticals. Ann ICRP. 1987;18:1–4.
11. Stabin MG, Sparks RB, Crowe E. OLINDA/EXM: the second-generation personal computer software for internal dose assessment in nuclear medicine. J Nucl Med. 2005;46(6):1023–7. 46/6/1023 [pii].
12. Klett R, Puille M, Matter HP, Steiner D, Sturz H, Bauer R. Activity leakage and radiation exposure in radiation synovectomy of the knee: influence of different therapeutic modalities. Z Rheumatol. 1999;58(4):207–12.
13. Stabin MG, Eckerman KF, Ryman JC, Williams LE. Bremsstrahlung radiation dose in yttrium-90 therapy applications. J Nucl Med. 1994;35(8):1377–80.

Radiation Exposure of Medical Staff and Radiation Protection Measures

Ilona Barth and Arndt Rimpler

Contents

8.1 Introduction

Radiosynoviorthesis (RSO) requires the use of unsealed radioactive sources in the form of radionuclide solutions or colloidal suspensions.

The three common RSO nuclides, Yttrium-90, Erbium-169 and Rhenium-186 emit beta (β^-) particles. Y-90 and Er-169 are pure beta emitters, whereas Re-186 also produces gamma radiation in 12 % of the decays. Relevant physical and radiological parameters of these nuclides are listed in Table 8.1. For comparison, the data of the most frequently used nuclides for diagnostics, Tc-99 m, are also given.

Obviously, as can be derived from the last three columns of the table, the dose rate factors (dose rate per unit of activity) and, thus, the hazard of skin exposure of

I. Barth, Dipl-Biol (✉) • A. Rimpler, Dipl-Phys
Department of Radiation Protection and Health, Federal Office for Radiation Protection (BfS), Koepenicker Allee 120 – 130, Berlin 10318, Germany
e-mail: ibarth@bfs.de

© Springer International Publishing Switzerland 2015
W.U. Kampen, M. Fischer (eds.), *Local Treatment of Inflammatory Joint Diseases: Benefits and Risks*, DOI 10.1007/978-3-319-16949-1_8

Table 8.1 Relevant data of RSO nuclides in comparison with Tc-99 m [1]

Nuclide	Radiation type	$T_{1/2}$	$E_{\beta.max}$ [keV]	p [%]	$E\gamma$ [keV]	p [%]	Maximum beta range in plastic [mm]	Dose rate factor[a] [mSv/hGBq]		Contact with 5 ml syringe[b]	[mSv/h] Contamination of 1 MBq in 0.05 ml droplet
								30 cm from point source			
Y-90	β-	2.67 days	2,284	100	–	–	9.2	108	–	43,500	1,350
Re-186	β-/γ	3.78 days	1,077	72	137	9	3.4	120	0.04	380	910
			939	22	59	3					
Er-169	β-	9.40 days	352	58	–	–	0.8	9.2	–	<<[c]	280
			344	42							
Tc-99 m	γ	6.01 h	120[d]	9	141	89	0.3	–	0.26	354	9

$T_{1/2}$ half-life, $E_{\beta.max}$ maximum beta energy, E_γ gamma energy, p emission probability

[a]First column: skin dose rate, second column: deep tissue dose rate

[b]On 1 ml syringes, the dose rate is higher because of lower self-shielding

[c]Only very low dose rate due to bremsstrahlung

[d]Internal conversion electrons

staff members are much higher for beta particles than for gammas and also depends strongly on the maximum beta energy.

In situations of low radiation protection standards, the medical staff may receive high exposures (mainly to the skin on their hands) that might exceed the annual skin dose limit of 500 mSv [2]. Therefore, appropriate safety standards have to be strictly complied with.

8.2   General Radiation Protection Principles

Radiation protection is based on three rationales: justification, limitation and optimisation. These principles are defined and elucidated in numerous international recommendations (e.g. IAEA 1996 [3]) and national regulations. Particularly, the International Commission on Radiological Protection (ICRP) has addressed the nuclear medical community with several publications focusing on radiation protection of staff and patients in general and nuclear medicine [4–8]. In addition, the International Atomic Energy Agency (IAEA) has issued some comprehensive publications on this topic [9–11]. In the European Union, the basic safety standards for protection against the dangers arising from exposure to ionising radiation were implemented in the Council Directive 2013/59/ Euratom (2013) [12].

8.2.1   Justification

A general definition of the justification principle is given in the European basic safety standards: "Medical exposure shall show a sufficient net benefit, weighing the total potential diagnostic or therapeutic benefits it produces, including the direct benefits to health of an individual and the benefits to society, against the individual detriment that the exposure might cause, taking into account the efficacy, benefits and risks of available alternative techniques having the same objective but involving no or less exposure to ionising radiation" [12]. In the EANM procedure guidelines for radiosynovectomy (2003) [13] and in Mödder (1995) [14], general justification criteria for RSO are given.

In the context of this article, the justification, i.e. the individual medical indication for a radionuclide therapy, is taken for granted and shall not be discussed here; however, it is a further precondition also for the justification of the occupational exposure of medical staff.

8.2.2   Limitation

The ICRP has defined dose limits for workers, which have been implemented in most countries [15].

The limit on the effective dose for occupational exposure shall be 20 mSv in any single year. However, in special circumstances or for certain exposure situations specified in national legislation, a higher effective dose of up to 50 mSv may be authorised by the competent authority in a single year, provided that the average annual dose over any five consecutive years – including the years for which the limit has been exceeded – does not exceed 20 mSv.

In most countries, the limit on the equivalent dose for the eye lens is still defined as 150 mSv in national legislation, but ICRP (2011) [16] and EURATOM (2013) [12] recommend 20 mSv in a single year or 100 mSv in any five consecutive years (subject to a maximum dose of 50 mSv in a single year).

In addition to the limits on effective dose, several limits on equivalent dose shall apply.

Especially in nuclear medicine, the limit on the equivalent skin dose (500 mSv per year) is of specific concern. In this case, the dose shall be averaged over an area of 1 cm^2, regardless of the area exposed. For keeping the limit, the area considered is that where the highest dose is suggested.

For pregnant and breastfeeding workers, the equivalent dose to the unborn child shall be as low as reasonably achievable and unlikely to exceed 1 mSv during at least the remainder of the pregnancy after pregnancy has been notified to the employer. These members of staff shall not do work which involves a significant risk of intake of radionuclides or bodily contamination.

For apprentices aged between 16 and 18 years and for students aged between 16 and 18 years who, in the course of their studies, have to work with radiation sources, the limit on their effective dose shall be 6 mSv in a year. The equivalent dose limit for the eye lens shall be 15 mSv and for the skin, for extremities, 150 mSv in a year, respectively.

For emergency situations, the occupational exposure limit shall be set, in general, below an effective dose of 100 mSv. In exceptional situations, in order to save lives, prevent severe radiation-induced health effects or prevent the development of catastrophic conditions, a reference level for the effective dose from external radiation of emergency workers may be set above 100 mSv but no higher than 500 mSv. Before they start working, the workers must be informed clearly and comprehensively about the associated health risks and the available protection measures. They undertake these actions voluntarily.

8.2.3   Optimisation

To make sure that a worker does not receive or exceed the dose limits, all procedures that may cause exposures of staff members have to be optimised regarding radiation protection. The most common rule of optimisation in radiation protection is the "ALARA principle". The acronym refers to the principle of keeping radiation doses "as low as reasonably achievable". In this context, economic aspects, i.e. the costs of protection measures, should be taken into account.

8.3 Radiation Protection Measures

8.3.1 Shielding

Shielding is a very effective protection measure, and it should be a matter of course that appropriate shielding for vials and syringes are used in everyday nuclear medicine and radiopharmacy operations. Materials with high density, i.e. with high atomic numbers Z, such as tungsten or lead are most suitable for the protection against gamma radiation. Generally, these shields are also appropriate for mixed beta/gamma emitters, for example, Re-186. However, its larger weight makes handling difficult. Therefore, shields from low-Z materials, e.g. transparent plastic such as acrylic glass or polycarbonate, are preferred for radionuclides that emit high-energy betas, such as Y-90 and Re-186. Besides, the use of low-Z shields minimises secondary bremsstrahlung. Though, it should be mentioned that the contribution of bremsstrahlung to the (total) exposure is often overestimated, and top priority is given to the efficient shielding of the betas. Monte Carlo simulations showed that Y-90 is shielded more effectively by 5 mm tungsten than by 10 mm acrylic glass because of the additional absorption of the bremsstrahlung [17]. This, however, is only important when high activities must be shielded and is not relevant for RSO.

The shielding thickness required depends on nuclide type and the activity. Moreover, a syringe shield should have a manageable size and weight. Beta particles are completely absorbed if the thickness of the shielding material exceeds the maximum particle range (see Table 8.1). For Y-90 ($E_{\beta,max} = 2.3$ MeV), the nuclide with the highest beta energy used in nuclear medicine, the range in plastic is about 9 mm. Therefore, shields that are designed for Y-90 are also appropriate for Re-186 ($E_{\beta,max} = 1.08$ MeV), which has a maximum range of 3.4 mm. Handling of Er-169 does not require vial or syringe shields. Their low-energy beta particles ($E_{\beta,max} = 0.35$ MeV) have a short range (plastic: 0.8 mm, glass: 0.5 mm), and they are not able to penetrate the walls of common syringes or vials. The dose rate is additionally decreased due to the self-shielding within the radionuclide solution. Further attenuation of the exposure is provided by protective gloves.

There are several types of shields for vials, syringes and containers available that are used for therapeutic radiopharmaceuticals. Most of them are also appropriate for beta emitters and should also be employed for RSO procedures. Figure 8.1 shows a typical syringe shield designed especially for the 1 ml syringes common in RSO.

However, the use of suitable shielding does not guarantee tolerable radiation exposures. Even when applying a syringe shield, there is still an unshielded area with high dose rates at its base. In particular, during the injection of the nuclides into the joints, the needle has to be placed carefully in the joint. Usually, the needle hub is fixed with two fingers during the injection for some seconds. This common practice, during which the almost unshielded finger tips are in close contact with the Y-90 activity, may cause very high local skin exposures within a short period of time. To avoid this, a special protective ring has been developed. It provides both

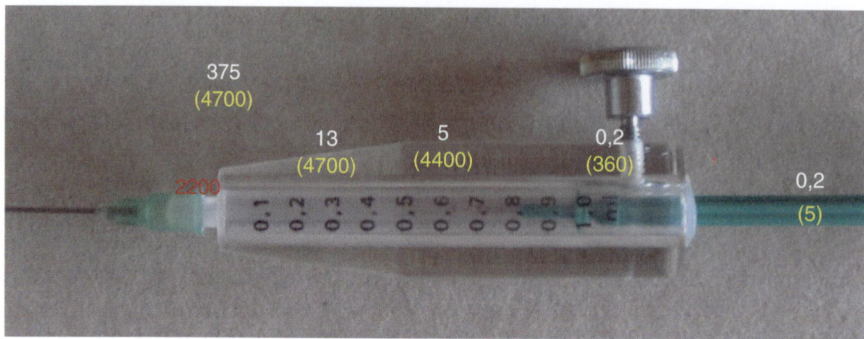

Fig. 8.1 Impact of an acrylic shield on the dose rate (μSv/s) around a Y-90 syringe containing 185 MBq Y-90. In *brackets*: dose rate without shielding

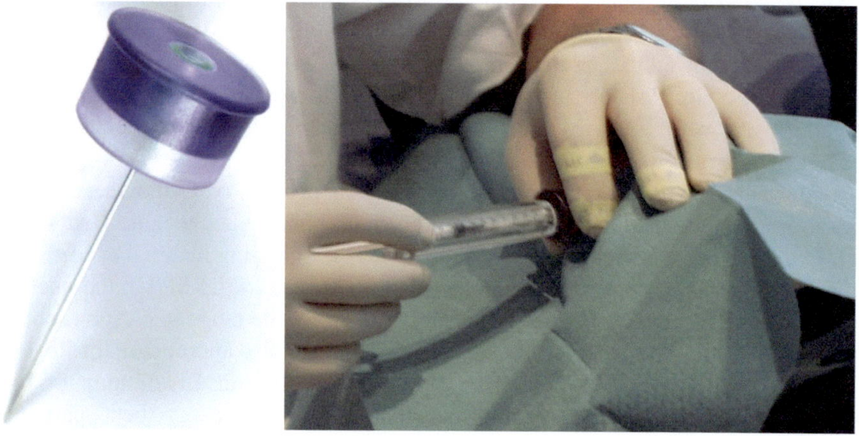

Fig. 8.2 One-way Macrolonring™ connected to a needle; available commercially from IBA Molecular (*left*); use of the Macrolonring™ during an injection of Y-90 into the knee (*right*)

shielding and distance to the needle. This Macrolonring™ (Fig. 8.2) is available in sterile packages. It fits to Braun-type needles only and must be put over the needle before performing the puncture. The ring should also be used to reduce skin exposure during the preparation of active syringes (Fig. 8.3).

Of course, shields often hamper handling, especially when injecting the radiopharmaceutical into the joint. However, it is wrong to believe that shielding might as well be ignored if only you work faster. An acrylic shielding reduces the dose rate by one or two orders of magnitude. In contrast, it is impossible to increase your working speed by such a factor.

The whole body and eye exposure of staff during preparation can be reduced significantly when the withdrawal of syringes is performed behind conventional bench top shields such as lead walls, castles or lead glass windows. RSO staff can also protect themselves against beta radiation by means of special commercially available or "home-made" acrylic benchtop shields.

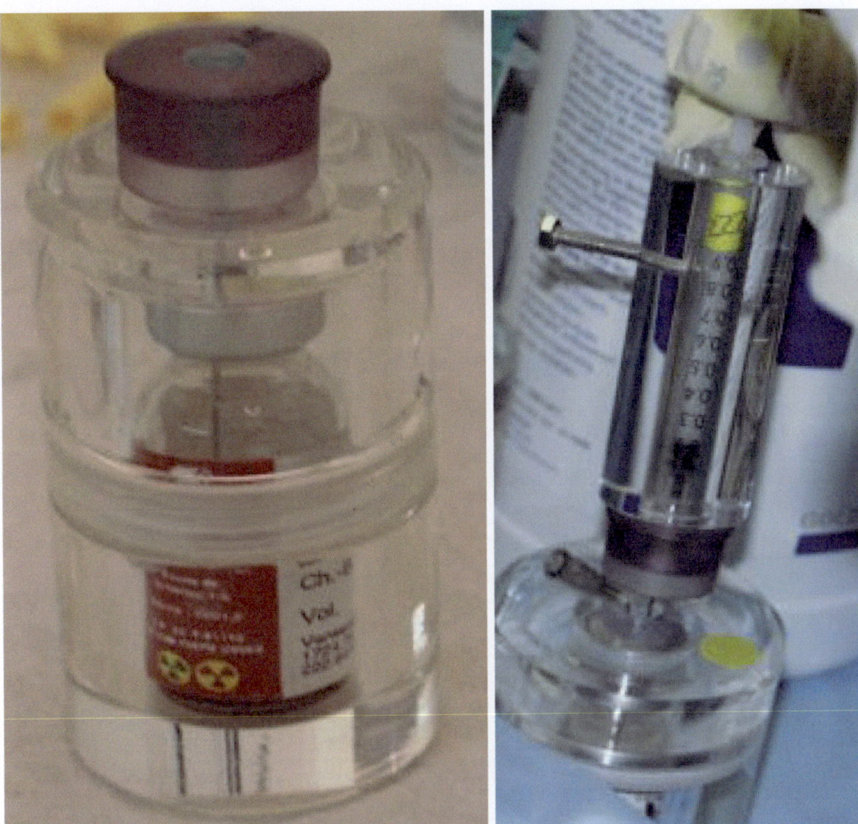

Fig. 8.3 Use of a Macrolonring™ during withdrawal of the syringes

The syringes filled with radiopharmaceuticals should be stored and transported to the treatment room in an acrylic glass box (Fig. 8.4) or, alternatively, in a common glass tray with a lid.

Due to the fact that used and apparently empty needles, syringes, vials, etc. may contain considerable amounts of radionuclides, waste containers also have to be shielded adequately.

When manipulating nuclides that emit high-energy betas – such as Y-90 – exposure of the eye lens must also be taken into consideration.

8.3.2   Distance

Even experienced radiopharmaceutical or clinical staff often does not know that the high-energy betas from Y-90 have a maximum range of about 9 m in air. However, it should be well established that good enough, the dose rate decreases with the square of the distance to the source. Therefore, keeping the distance is the easiest and cheapest measure in terms of radiation protection, and all

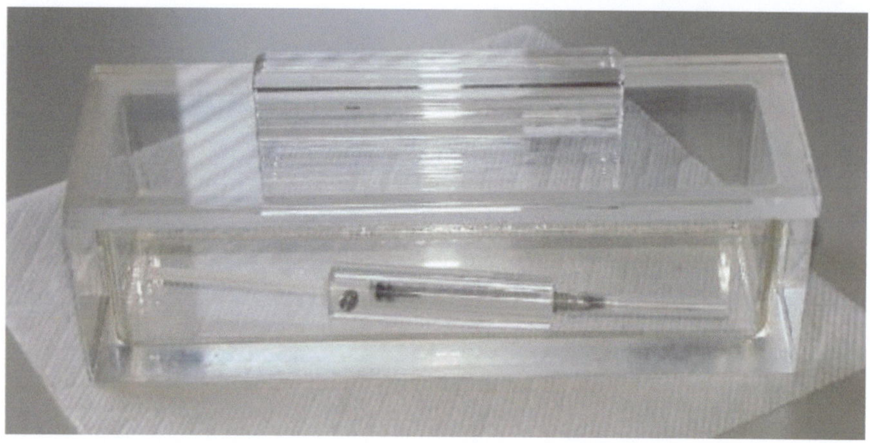

Fig. 8.4 Transport and storage box made of acrylic glass

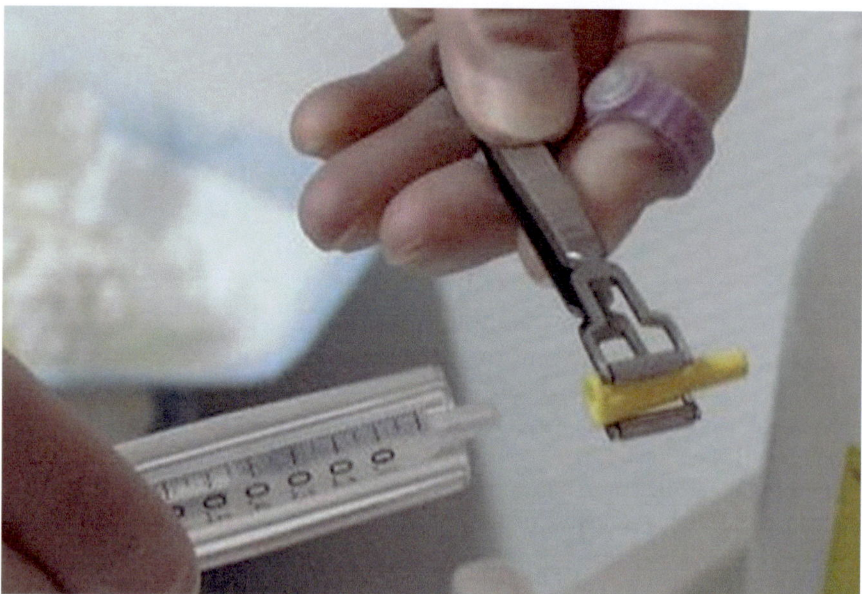

Fig. 8.5 Special forceps for plugs

opportunities should be used to take advantage of the distance to radioactive substances. This is especially important in all situations where the processing of unshielded radiopharmaceuticals cannot be avoided. In such situations, the use of tools (such as clamps and pincers), which also diminish the risk of skin contamination, is strongly recommended. Figures 8.5 and 8.6 exemplify the use of such tools in RSO.

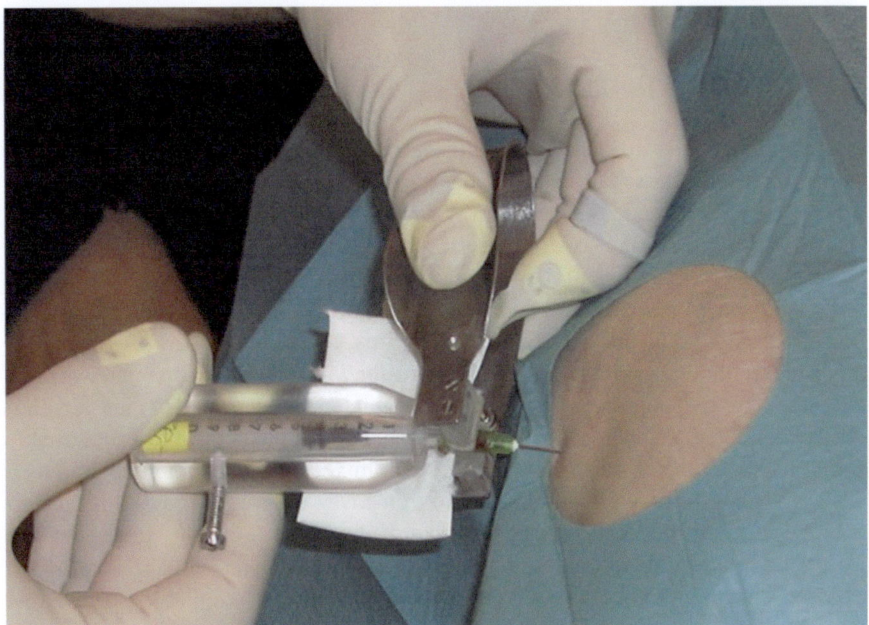

Fig. 8.6 Special forceps used for holding the needle during injection

The principle to never make direct contact with unshielded vessels containing radionuclides with your fingers should be observed. This also holds true for any potentially contaminated vessels such as vials, syringes, tubes, etc. after discharging a radioactive liquid. The remaining activity within apparently empty vessels may be in the order of some 10 MBq, and careless direct contact to the skin may result in unnecessarily high exposures. Therefore, shielding and keeping your distance should also be considered when disposing of contaminated material and radioactive waste. Adequate waste management and disposal are a special task that cannot be discussed here in detail. IAEA (2006) [10], for example, gives additional advice.

Admittedly, there is a high degree of dexterity necessary in order to inject a solution into a joint using forceps, instead of gripping the needle with a hand. Moreover, the risk for injection outside of the joint increases. This practice requires special training. Alternatively, the above-mentioned Macrolonring™ should be used (Fig. 8.2).

Moreover, when manipulating beta-emitting nuclides with high-energy, e.g. Y-90, exposure of the eye lens must also be taken into consideration, especially against the background of the recent ICRP (2011) [16] recommendation to reduce the annual dose limit to the eye lens from 150 to 20 mSv. The use of shielding and increasing the distance also improve the protection of the eye lens. For answering the question of whether wearing protective glasses in the field of RSO is necessary, studies are still in progress.

8.4   Monitoring

8.4.1   Personal Dosimetry

Nuclear medicine staff must be routinely monitored for occupational radiation exposure, both to their whole body and parts of their bodies, if 3/10 of the dose limits might be exceeded, e.g. 150 mSv for the skin dose. Commonly, a personal dosimeter for monitoring the effective dose is worn on the chest, usually with film, thermoluminescence (TLD) or optically stimulated luminescence (OSL) dosimeters. It is also recommended to wear an additional extremity dosimeter for monitoring the skin dose to the hands for the majority of radiation workers in nuclear medicine, including radiopharmacy staff. Mostly TLD ring dosimeters are worn on the fingers for this purpose. Usually, these dosimeters are designed to measure photon radiation, e.g. in interventional radiology. In nuclear medicine, the more suitable solution is to wear ring dosimeters designed for mixed beta and photon fields. These dosimeters consist of a special TLD with a thin cover. Figure 8.7 shows three different types of these well-established dosimeters.

Even if appropriate individual dosimeters are available and actually worn by the exposed staff, monitoring does not necessarily provide results suitable to prove that the skin dose limit is observed. There is another essential issue to be considered: when handling radiopharmaceuticals in medical practices, staff in particular is exposed to rather non-uniform radiation fields. It is advisable to measure the skin dose at the part of the body which presumably receives the highest exposure.

The problem of valid skin dose monitoring was subject of the European research project ORAMED ("optimisation of radiation protection for medical staff") [17]. Measurements of individual doses and their distribution across the hands of staff were performed in nuclear medicine diagnostics and therapy. This extensive study confirmed earlier results from RSO [2] as well as from other fields of nuclear

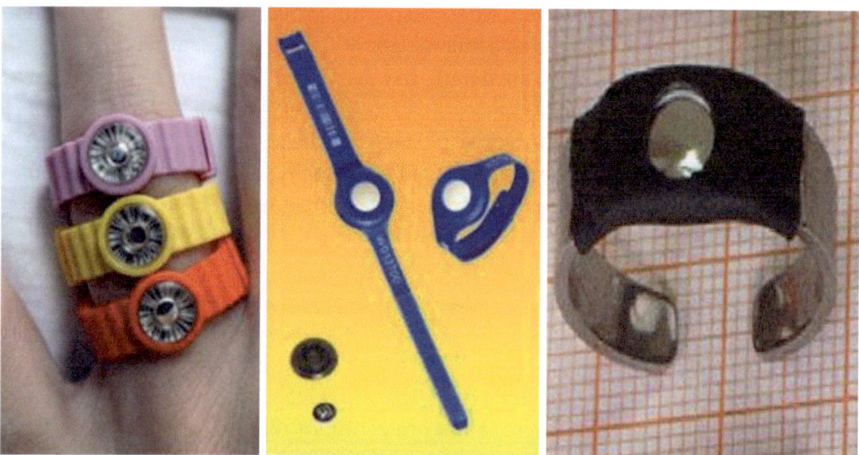

Fig. 8.7 Different types of ring dosimeters

medicine [18]: the thumb or index finger tips on the nondominant hand most frequently receives the highest dose [19].

Since the fingertip is not suited to wear a ring dosimeter, it should be worn preferably on the index finger base (first phalanx) of the nondominant hand, with the detector turned to the palmar direction [20]. The dosimeters should not be worn on the ring finger of the dominant hand, as it is common.

However, even if the routine ring dosimeter is attached to the base of the nondominant hand's index finger, the maximum skin dose is underestimated by a factor of about 6 on average. This factor increases considerably when wearing the dosimeter, e.g. on the ring finger or on the wrong hand. The deviation between the dosimeter reading and the maximum dose also increases when the radiation field is more inhomogeneous, e.g. due to insufficient protection measures, such as working without shields. Routine skin dose monitoring often results in severe underestimation of actual skin exposure and, consequently, in a belittlement of the hazard. Therefore, more effort has to be put into improving radiation protection measures.

8.4.2 Contamination Monitoring

Since RSO requires the handling of unsealed liquid radionuclides, there is an increased risk of skin contamination and incorporation. It goes without saying that eating, drinking and smoking are prohibited in controlled areas.

Nitrile or vinyl instead of latex gloves should be worn to avoid hand contamination, since some radioactive solutions may easily penetrate latex. Before leaving the controlled area, hands have to be routinely checked for contamination with an appropriate contamination monitor that should be in stand-by mode in any nuclear medical facility. The responsible staff members must be trained both in performing measurements of contamination measurements and in decontamination measures.

More detailed instructions related to radiation protection in radionuclide therapy are given in IAEA (2006) [10]. Advice that is particularly useful for several radionuclides is also available on a number of websites, among them the American Health Physics Society's (HPS) [21] homepage.

References

1. Delacroix D, Guerre JP, Leblanc P, et al. Radionuclide and radiation protection data handbook 2002. Radiat Prot Dosim. 2002;98:1.
2. Barth I, Mielcarek J. Occupational exposure during radiosynoviorthesis. In: Proceedings of the 6th European ALARA Network Workshop "Occupational Exposure Optimisation in the Medical Field and Radiopharmaceutical Industry." Madrid, 23–25 Oct 2002. p. 43–6, ISBN 84-7834-437-3.
3. IAEA. International basis safety standards for protection against ionizing radiation and for the safety of radioactive sources, IAEA Safety Series, vol. 115. Vienna: International Atomic Energy Agency; 1996. PO Box 100, A-1400.
4. ICRP. Radiological protection and safety in medicine. International Commission on Radiological Protection, Publication 73, Ann. ICRP vol 26(2). Oxford: Elsevier; 1996.

5. ICRP. International Commission on Radiological Protection radiation dose to patients from radiopharmaceuticals, Publication 80, Ann. ICRP vol 28(3). Oxford: Elsevier; 1998.
6. ICRP. International Commission on Radiological Protection pregnancy and medical radiation, Publication 84, Ann. ICRP vol 30(1). Oxford: Elsevier; 2000.
7. ICRP. International Commission on Radiological Protection release of patients after therapy with unsealed radionuclides, Publication 94, Ann. ICRP vol 34(2). Oxford: Elsevier; 2004.
8. ICRP. International Commission on Radiological Protection, the 2007 recommendations of the International commission on radiological protection, ICRP Publication 103, Ann. ICRP 37(2–4). Oxford: Elsevier; 2007.
9. IAEA. International Atomic Energy Agency, applying radiation safety standards in nuclear medicine. IAEA Safety Report Series No. 40, Vienna. 2005.
10. IAEA. International Atomic Energy Agency, nuclear medicine resources manual. Vienna: International Atomic Energy Agency; 2006. ISBN 92-0-107504-9.
11. IAEA. International Atomic Energy Agency, release of patients after radionuclide therapy. Safety Report Series No. 63, Vienna. 2009.
12. EURATOM. 2013. COUNCIL DIRECTIVE 2013/59/EURATOM of 5 Dec 2013 laying down basic safety standards for protection against the dangers arising from exposure to ionising radiation, and repealing Directives 89/618/Euratom, 90/641/Euratom, 96/29/Euratom, 97/43/Euratom and 2003/122/Euratom, EN Off J Eur Union 14.01.2013, L13/1ff.
13. EANM Procedure Guidelines for Radiosynovectomy. EANM procedure guidelines for radiosynovectomy. Eur J Nucl Med. 2003;30(3):BP16. March 2003 – EANM 2003.
14. Mödder G. Radiosynoviorthesis: involvement of nuclear medicine in rheumatology and orthopaedics. Mecckenheim: Warlich; 1995.
15. ICRP. International Commission on Radiological Protection general principles for the radiation protection of workers, Publication 75, Ann. ICRP vol 27(1). Oxford: Elsevier; 1997.
16. ICRP. International Commission on Radiological Protection, statement on tissue reactions. 21 Apr 2011.
17. ORAMED. 2011. http://www.oramed-fp7.eu/.
18. Whitby M, Martin CJ. A multi-centre study of dispensing methods and hand doses in UK hospital radiopharmacies. Nucl Med Commun. 2005;26:49–60.
19. Rimpler A, Barth I, Ferrari P, et al. Extremity exposure in nuclear medicine therapy with 90Y-labelled substances – Results of the ORAMED project. to be published in Rad Meas. (2011). http://dx.doi.org/10.1016/j.radmeas.2011.05.068.
20. Sans Merce M, Ruiz N, Barth I, et al. Recommendations to reduce hand exposure for standard nuclear medicine procedures. Radiat Meas. 2011;46:1330–3.
21. HPS http://hpschapters.org/northcarolina/nuclide_information_library.php3.

Local Complications After Radiosynovectomy and Possible Treatment Strategies: A Literature Survey

9

Willm Uwe Kampen

Contents

9.1   Introduction

Radiosynovectomy (RSO) is performed by intra-articular injection of three different radiocolloids, normally guided by fluoroscopy; the radiopharmaceuticals are phagocytized by the synovial lining cells leading to a radiogenic sclerosis and fibrosis of the inflamed synovial membrane and thus to a significant reduction of joint effusion and pain. Apart from unavoidable systemic side effects like the low whole-body radiation load and a transient flush associated with coadministered intra-articular corticosteroids, possible serious local side effects or complications after radiosynovectomy are:

1. Superficial skin or needle track ulceration
2. Radionecrosis of the juxta-articular soft tissue
3. Intra-articular infection
4. Thromboembolic complications due to posttreatment joint immobilization

W.U. Kampen
Nuklearmedizin Spitalerhof, Spitalerstr. 8, Hamburg 20095, Germany
e-mail: kampen@nuklearmedizin-spitalerhof.de

© Springer International Publishing Switzerland 2015
W.U. Kampen, M. Fischer (eds.), *Local Treatment of Inflammatory Joint Diseases: Benefits and Risks*, DOI 10.1007/978-3-319-16949-1_9

Most of these side effects are preventable if the injection is carefully done under aseptic conditions, if the intra-articular needle placement is secured, and if the correct radionuclide in an appropriate activity is chosen for therapy. However, some cases are documented in the literature and should be discussed in this chapter.

9.2   Radiogenic Tissue Damage of Different Severity

Local skin and needle track ulceration or even severe necrosis of periarticular soft tissues are the most serious complications of radiosynovectomy. A reflux of the radiocolloid during retraction of the needle with concomitant deposition of a small amount of activity in the subcutaneous tissues is probably the most frequent reason for superficial skin lesions or a so-called needle track ulceration. In a retrospective study covering 83 RSO procedures in 45 patients, 1 local skin lesion was documented [1]. Ruotsi et al. described "bullous eruptions" in two finger joints 3 weeks after RSO and one case of a "slight erythema" after 1 month in a total of 83 finger joints treated with Er-169 colloid [2]. Another case of a local skin necrosis was described at the site of injection of Y-90 colloid in a patient with severe bone destruction [3]. However, no details are mentioned on the need of a special treatment or the clinical course in these cases.

The author has observed one case of local skin redness and pain after treatment of a hip joint with 150 MBq Re-186 colloid which occurred 2 days after RSO. The distribution scan showed no abnormality and, thus, there was not a fear of a severe necrosis of deeper tissue layers. The symptoms regressed over a period of 3 weeks under increased resting and frequent local cooling using ice packs (see Fig. 9.1).

Savaser and colleagues reported a case of needle track ulceration after RSO of an ankle joint with Re-186 in 1999 [4]. The lesion showed scarred healing after a few weeks without any further treatment. In a series of 38 knee joints treated with Yttrium-90, three patients showed "minor pigmentation at the injection site"; a needle track ulceration was documented in two other patients [5] which required treatment with skin grafting in one case.

While superficial lesions often show (scarred) healing without any special therapy, larger necroses with radiogenic damage of deeper tissue layers should be promptly treated to shorten the course of the disease and to minimize the complaints of the respective patients. Necrosis of para-articular tissue by accidental para-articular injection of the radionuclide is indeed the worst local complication after radiosynovectomy. Due to a restricted blood supply of the necrotic area, the healing process is additionally hampered by a low oxygen content.

The frequency of larger skin or soft tissue necroses is generally assumed to be very low which is proven by the analysis of the periodic safety update reports (see chapter by Fischer et al. in this book). Two necroses from a total of 11,000 RSO procedures were reported by Kolarz and Thumb in 1982 [6]. In another study which involved interrogation of both 260 nuclear medicine physicians performing radiosynovectomy throughout Germany and 20 insurance companies engaged in medical liability using a standardized questionnaire and covering 5 years, a total of

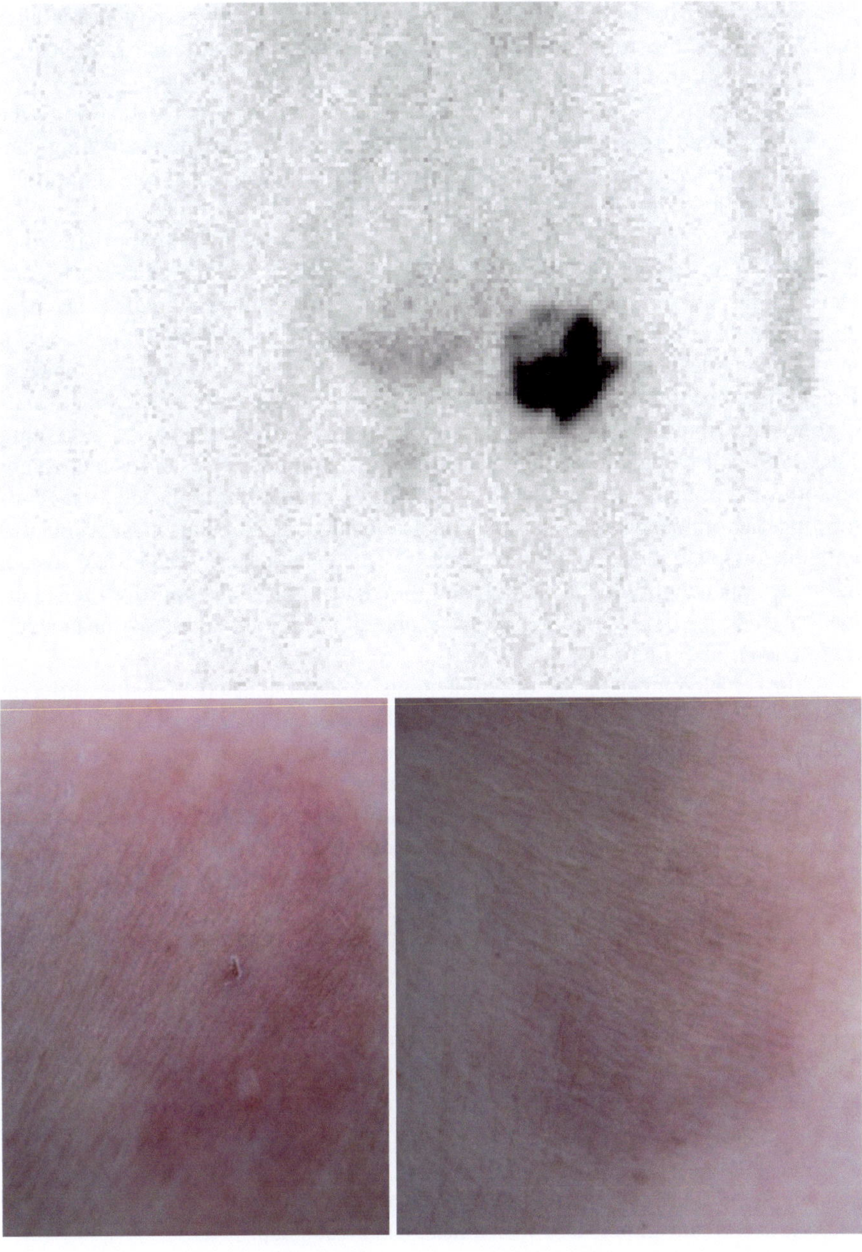

Fig. 9.1 Distribution scan after injection of 150 MBq Re-186-colloid into the left hip joint. *Lower left*: Circumscribed redness of the skin with a small moistened blain at the site of puncture 4 days after therapy. *Lower right*: Considerable fading of inflammatory activity 10 days after RSO, central defect is completely closed without any secretion

29 necroses were documented [7]. However, the response rate was only 25.7 % after 9 months. Thus, the true number of radionecroses after para-articular radionuclide application is probably higher but will never be reliably documented.

Deeper skin necroses have been documented in case reports [8, 9]. Due to the more pronounced deterioration of deeper tissue layers, a spontaneous healing cannot be expected, and surgical debridement and closure of the defect by skin grafting seems to be the adequate treatment.

Besides an insufficient injection technique, the choice of an inappropriate radionuclide and/or an excessive activity may be the reason for a radionecrosis. The choice of the appropriate radionuclide for a joint depends mainly on the tissue penetration depth of the beta particles which is particularly dependent on the energy of the radionuclide. This penetration depth must be suitable for the size of the joint which should be treated. Yttrium-90 has a maximum beta energy of 2.2 MeV resulting in a maximum tissue penetration depth up to 11 mm (mean value 3.6 mm). Thus, Y-90 is expected to be the most hazardous radionuclide used for radiosynovectomy and is approved for treatment of the knee joint only. Small joints (finger or toe joints, acromioclavicular, sternoclavicular, temporomandibular) must be injected with the low-energy beta emitter Erbium-169 (mean beta energy 0.34 MeV) which has a mean penetration depth of only 0.3 mm. Rhenium-186 is approved for treatment of mid-sized joints like wrist, elbow, ankle, or hip joint and has a mean penetration depth of 1.2 mm.

A further alignment to the different joints is accomplished by using different activities for joints of different sizes. This is documented in both national and international guidelines for radiosynovectomy, although not a legal requirement [10, 11].

Examples of radiogenic damage of the surrounding soft tissue following inappropriate choice of a radionuclide with an energy too high for the treated joint are published in the literature. Two necroses from RSO using Yttrium-90 in finger joints (metacarpophalangeal joint and proximal interphalangeal joint) were documented in an old study from 1972, covering a total of 250 treatment sessions [12]. However, no further information on the clinical course or treatment modalities is given in this paper. More recent studies showed severe complications with large, deep tissue ulcerations in ankle joints treated with Yttrium-90. Two cases of severe necroses were seen in a series of 7 RSO procedures of ankle joints treated with 555 MBq Yttrium-90 [13]. Another case report showed the same complication after RSO using Yttrium-90 in an ankle joint; however, the injected activity is not documented in this publication [14]. Thus, the combination of the "wrong" radionuclide (Yttrium-90 instead of Rhenium-186) and an excessive activity led to these serious complications which needed aggressive treatment with surgical excision of the necrotic soft tissue and closure with a fasciocutaneous flap.

The treatment of choice for these complications is still under debate. Some advice may be gained from therapy of radiogenic lesions after external beam radiation therapy. The common problem in both clinical settings is that radiation leads to parenchymal stem cell and vascular damage. This results in a reduced capacity of tissue regeneration from local hypoxia, finally leading to tissue necrosis [15]. Apart from a "wait-and-see" strategy or local conservative treatment, hyperbaric oxygen therapy may be used to overcome the local oxygen shortage. The higher oxygen partial pressure induces revascularization of irradiated tissue and thus promotes its self-healing mechanisms [16] with clinical success rates up to 93 % in treatment of radiation-induced edema, ulceration, and bone necroses [15]. In our own survey, hyperbaric oxygen therapy was used in three cases of tissue necrosis after para-articular injection of Re-186 colloid with clinical success in two of them. However, in one patient with a local radiogenic tissue defect from Yttrium-90, 40 sessions of hyperbaric oxygen did not prevent tissue necrosis, and surgical therapy was needed [7].

Successful treatment requires complete resection of the damaged tissue with consecutive closure of the defect with well-vascularized, nonirradiated tissue. Depending on the severity and the dimensions of the local defect, either regional pedicled flaps or free-tissue transfer has been used [7, 9]. Despite appropriate surgery, complications with local wound dehiscence, seroma, or blood vessel thrombosis are seen, sometimes resulting in complete flap loss [17]. Due to the very low beta energy, skin ulcers from Er-169 colloids are likely to heal spontaneously with less pronounced tissue damage.

9.3   Intra-articular Infection

Joint infection is a severe complication which is not related to the radiopharmaceutical agent itself but might occur from any joint puncture performed either for diagnostic or therapeutic purposes. The individual risk for intra-articular infection depends on several predisposing factors, e.g., systemic inflammatory disease (rheumatoid arthritis), immunocompetence, ongoing pharmacotherapy, existence of joint replacement, and others. The frequency of joint infections after intra-articular injections is generally assumed to be very low and ranges from 1:3000 down to 1:100.000 [18]. In a survey covering 126.000 arthrographies, only three intra-articular infections were documented [19].

Apart from poor non-aseptic injection technique or contamination of the injected drug preparation, an infection may arise from bacterial infection of deeper tissue layers not eliminated by skin disinfection [20] or from hematogenous spread along the needle track [21].

Published data concerning joint infections after RSO are very rare. Three cases with intra-articular infection were documented in a very early paper by Menkes in 1979 [22], reviewing a total of >9,000 RSO procedures between 1969 and 1975. One case of a septic arthritis after repeated RSO was described by Taylor et al. [23] in a series of 121 knee joint treatments using Yttrium-90. However, there is no further information about any treatment strategy or the clinical course of such complication.

In our data pool [7], a total of 13 intra-articular infections were documented. In seven of these patients, oral antibiotics did not lead to restitution and, thus, intra-articular antibiotics were needed. An endoscopic joint lavage was performed in four additional patients.

In our experience, two patients developed severe pain and massive joint swelling with redness and skin hyperthermia a few hours after treatment with RSO for chronic effusion after endoprosthetic knee joint replacement. As the clinical symptoms were typical for joint infection, the patients were immediately treated with oral antibiotics (fixed combination of amoxicillin 875 mg and clavulanate 125 mg twice a day) and showed complete regression of complaints and symptoms after 3 weeks.

Early and intense therapy is necessary in case of septic arthritis to prevent severe joint damage and ankylosis or even systemic complications. According to the guidelines, aspiration of joint fluid must be done if an intra-articular infection is suspected. This is mandatory for establishing the diagnosis and the choice of an appropriate pharmacotherapy according to the antibiogram. If the symptoms increase within 24–48 h or if repeated aspiration is unsuccessful, surgical treatment is indicated [24]. An early ("primary") surgical therapy was also recommended in the literature [25]. A lower intra-articular bacterial count rate, the clinical decompression after joint lavage, and the avoidance of a possible "non-responding" to the antibiotic treatment are possible advantages compared to the primary antibiotic therapy.

9.4   Thromboembolic Complications

As with intra-articular infections, thromboembolic complications are not specific for radionuclide joint treatment but may occur following the mandatory immobilization of the treated joint using a tight bandage and a splint. This holds especially true for radiosynovectomy of lower limb joints in old and immobile patients or for those with a concomitant high risk of thrombosis, e.g., varicose veins or coagulopathies for any reasons. However, there are no documented cases of a thromboembolic complication in the literature so far, which is definitely linked to the radiosynovectomy procedure.

In our survey, a total of 12 cases of thrombosis after radiosynovectomy of lower limb joints were documented: 1 of them after treatment of both the knee and the hip joint in the same patient. An elevated risk profile was documented in 6 of 12 patients, and no prophylactic anticoagulation was performed. Most of these patients (8/12) were successfully treated with routine anticoagulation pharmacotherapy. A guideline for effective treatment of venous thromboembolic disease recommends short-term treatment with subcutaneous low-molecular-weight heparin or unfractionated heparin given intravenously [26].

Provided there are no preexisting risk factors in the individual patient, the risk of a thromboembolic complication must be carefully weighed against possible side effects from anticoagulation therapy, and thus, a general thromboembolic prophylaxis cannot be recommended. If RSO is performed in two adjacent joints of the lower limb (knee and hip joint or knee and ankle joint), the immobilization of both joints leads to an increased ("medium") risk with 10–20 % deep venous thromboses of the shank, 2–4 % of more proximal thromboses, 1–2 % of clinically relevant pulmonary embolism, and 0.1–0.4 % of lethal pulmonary embolism [27]. In such patients and in those with two or more predisposing risk factors, an effective antithrombotic prophylaxis is mandatory [28]. Ready-to-use syringes containing low molecular heparin should be used for this purpose if the respective patient does not display any contraindications like bleeding abnormalities and cerebral or dissected aortic aneurysms.

9.5   Other Possible Complications: A Critical Review

Other complications published in the literature which are not direct results of RSO procedure and of minor severity include a transient and frequently self-limiting radiogenic effusion which has been documented in 2 % of patients several hours after radionuclide instillation [29]. A co-injection of a corticosteroid during radiosynovectomy helps to avoid this adverse event in the vast majority of patients [30]. Probably due to a tight bandage after RSO with compression of the local nerves, a transient fibular nerve paresis and symptoms mimicking Sudeck's dystrophy and carpal tunnel syndrome were documented in our survey, but there was no information on the further clinical course. A case of a radiogenic dermatitis has been documented which was probably a result of extended fluoroscopy during radiosynovectomy in a severely destroyed joint [7].

In a recently published study, a very high rate of osteonecroses (ON) and joint infections was found after RSO in patients suffering from osteoarthritis [31], and the authors stated that radiosynovectomy might not be as safe as it has been described before. However, this paper contained several methodological flaws which could have led to potentially incomplete or misleading conclusions.

First of all, the selection of patients is highly questionable. Kisielinski evaluated only 93 patients with 161 RSOs from a total of 80.000 RSOs within 12 years. The conclusion in the publication was thus made on a very small subgroup of 93/80.000 treatments (0.2 %), and nothing is stated about the eligibility criteria. Out of these 93 patients, 22 (with 49 of 80.000 RSOs)=0.05 % suffered from ON and/or infection which is a very low rate of these serious events.

Most patients (50/79) had a Kellgren-Lawrence stage 4 with pronounced mutilations of the treated joint. Due to the considerably increased bone turnover in osteoarthritis, bone scanning cannot differentiate exactly between osteonecrosis and osteoarthritis if performed prior to RSO. To exclude preexisting osteonecrosis, a normal bone scan (or MRI) must be postulated but is never seen in patients with osteoarthritis in a Kellgren-Lawrence stage 3 and 4. In addition, osteonecrosis after RSO was diagnosed by methods with higher sensitivity and specificity (even intraoperatively or by histopathology). Therefore, it is not possible to point out whether osteonecrosis has developed after RSO or has been already present prior to RSO.

Osteonecrosis is a disease characterized by disturbance of local blood circulation but in many patients connected with several risk factors: cortisone for rheumatoid arthritis or COPD, cytostatics, abuse of alcohol and nicotine, trauma, irradiation, diabetes mellitus, and osteoporosis [32]. One main bias of the retrospective evaluation by Kisielinski et al. is the lack of a control group suffering from same risk factors. Franchi and Bullough [33] reported on 11.7 % avascular necroses in femoral heads removed because of osteoarthritis; in about 20 % of specimens with ON, there was evidence of microfractures in the trabecular bone. In the publication of Kisielinski et al., 13 of 22 patients suffering from ON were postmenopausal women, only 2 of them less than 60 years. The probability of osteoporosis in this group is quite high. In most patients included in this study, Kellgren Lawrence stage 4 disease was confirmed. By definition, stage 4 is characterized by an advanced narrowing up to total loss of the joint space; articular cartilage is destroyed widely. This may lead to a loss of functioning buffer capacity resulting in traumatic microfractures in these parts of the bone, especially in osteoporotic patients. Seven of them had additional risk factors (RA on continuous corticosteroid therapy, COPD, and/or diabetes mellitus) enhancing the risk of ON.

To judge the risk of radiation to the subchondral bone with possible induction of local osteonecroses, no exact data about radiation doses to bone surface are discussed. The calculated radiation dose to bone surface after RSO of the knee joint using Yttrium-90 was 27–30 Gy [34]. The threshold for causing ON is 30 Gy [35]. Höller et al. reported ON of the pelvis after irradiation dose exceeding 50 Gy in 14 % [36]. Thus, local radiation of the bone is a clear risk factor for osteonecrosis, but radiation dose to the bone surface in RSO with Yttrium-90 is below threshold and with Rhenium-186, far less.

The authors argued that intra-articular infection was caused by RSO in five patients. Infection following RSO was strongly correlated to arthroplasty with a high degree of significance. However, a possible "low-grade" infection was never excluded prior to RSO, especially in patients with total knee replacement (three of five). In 2009, Jämsen et al. [37] published an incidence of 0.9 % surgical revisions in a register-based analysis of 43,149 otherwise uncomplicated cases. Hyperglycemia is also known to be significantly associated with infected knee replacement [38].

In the publication of Kisielinski, there are no data given relative to clinical signs of infection in joints that showed a positive bacteriology. Especially in patients with proven *Staphylococcus epidermidis* and *S. oralis*, it seems possible that infection was caused by diagnostic puncture and not during RSO. Thus, a clear correlation between intra-articular infection and joint puncture during RSO is not proven by the authors.

In addition to RSO, the patients showed many other factors that may have cause a higher risk for osteonecrosis. Therefore, a multifactorial analysis should have been done. The authors simply used Spearman's rank test. This is a test to find correlations, but simple correlation gives no information about causality.

Therefore, in this retrospective study, it is not possible to conclude that RSO leads to osteonecrosis or infection. The general problem of any retrospective evaluation is the quality of data and how they can be controlled. In the publication of Kisielinski et al., a small number of patients with a large number of different variables are evaluated. Moreover, the variation of diagnostic procedures with different sensitivity and specificity prior to and after RSO confirming osteonecrosis probably is attributable to the quality of the study. The methodology used has significantly biased the presented results which should not be taken too seriously.

Conclusion

Radiosynoviorthesis is a safe local treatment option for patients suffering from inflammatory joint disease. However, appropriate patient selection, the choice of the correct radionuclide with an adequate activity for the respective joint, a skillful and aseptic injection technique, and a reasonable follow-up are indispensable to achieve a maximum of therapeutic efficacy with a minimum of possible hazards.

In case of any complications, the following *treatment recommendations* can be stated from literature data and own experiences:

- Any complaints of the patients must be taken for serious.
- Early surgical therapy with broad excision of the necrotic tissue and closure of the defect should be done in case of tissue damage from Yttrium-90.
- Hyperbaric oxygen therapy may be sufficient for treatment of Rhenium-186-induced ulcers. In case of therapeutic failure, surgery seems advisable.
- Lesions from Erbium-169 will probably heal by conservative treatment.
- Clinical signs of intra-articular infection after RSO should be secured by immediate fluid aspiration and bacterial culture. If an initial oral antibiotic treatment does not improve the situation significantly within 24–48 h, the infection should be treated by joint lavage or endoscopy together with the local application of intra-articular antibiotics.
- Prophylactic anticoagulation against thromboembolism from posttreatment immobilization is recommended only in patients after RSO of two adjacent joints of the lower limb and in patients with at least two risk factors.

References

1. Jahangier ZN, Jacobs JW, von Isselt JW, Bijlsma JW. Persistent synovitis treated with radiation synovectomy using yttrium-90: a retrospective evaluation of 83 procedures for 45 patients. Br J Rheumatol. 1997;36:861–9.
2. Ruotsi A, Hypen M, Rekonen A, Oka M. Erbium-169 versus triamcinolone hexacetonide in the treatment of rheumatoid finger joints. Ann Rheum Dis. 1979;38:45–7.
3. Molho P, Verrier P, Stieltjes N, Schacher JM, Ounnoughene N, Vassilieff D, Menkes CJ, Sultan Y. A retrospective study on chemical and radioactive synovectomy in severe haemophilia patients with recurrent haemarthrosis. Haemophilia. 1999;5:115–23.
4. Savaser AN, Hoffmann KT, Soerensen H, Banzer DH. Die Radiosynoviorthese im Behandlungsplan chronisch-entzündlicher Gelenkerkrankungen. Z Rheumatol. 1999;58:71–8.
5. Jacob R, Smith T, Prakasha B, Joannides T. Yttrium^{90} synovectomy in the management of chronic knee arthritis: a single institution experience. Rheumatol Int. 2003;23:216–20.
6. Kolarz G, Thumb N. Methods of nuclear medicine in rheumatology. Stuttgart: Schattauer-Verlag; 1982.
7. Kampen WU, Matis E, Czech N, Soti Z, Henze E. Serious complications after radiosynoviorthesis. Survey on frequency and treatment modalities. Nuklearmedizin. 2006;45(6):262–8.
8. Sojan S, Bartholomaeusz D. Cutaneous radiation necrosis as a complication of yttrium-90 synovectomy. Hell J Nucl Med. 2005;8:58–9.

9. Öztürk H, Öztemür Z, Bulut O. Treatment of skin necrosis after radiation synovectomy with yttrium-90: a case report. Rheumatol Int. 2008;28:1067–8.

10. Farahati J, Reiners C, Fischer M, Moedder G, Franke J, Mahlstedt J, Soerensen H. Guidelines for radiosynovectomy. Nuklearmed. 1999;38:254–5.

11. Clunie G, Fischer M, EANM. EANM procedure guidelines for radiosynovectomy. Eur J Nucl Med Mol Imaging. 2003;30:BP12–6.

12. Menkes CJ, Aignan M, Ingrand J, Lego A, Roucayrol JC, Belbarre F. La synoviorthese par les radio-isotopes a la main et au poignet. Rev Chir Orthop. 1972;58(59):432–9.

13. Bickels J, Isaakov J, Kollender Y, Meller I. Unacceptable complications following intra-articular injection of yttrium 90 in the ankle joint for diffuse pigmented villonodular synovitis. J Bone Joint Surg. 2008;90:326–8.

14. Peters W, Lee P. Radiation necrosis overlying ankle joint after injection with Yttrium-90. Ann Plast Surg. 1994;32:542–3.

15. Tibbles PM, Edelsberg JS. Hyperbaric oxygen therapy. N Engl J Med. 1996;334:1642–8.

16. Borg M, Wilkinson D, Humeniuk V, Norman J. Successful treatment of radiation induced breast ulcer with hyperbaric oxygen. Breast. 2001;10:336–41.

17. Guerlek A, Miller MJ, Amin AA, Evans GRD, Reece GP, Baldwin BJ, Schusterman MA, Kroll SS, Robb GL. Reconstruction of complex radiation-induced injuries using free-tissue transfer. J Reconstr Microsurg. 1998;14:337–40.

18. Holland C, Jaeger L, Smentkowski U, Weber B, Otto C. Septic and aseptic complications of corticosteroid injections. Dtsch Ärzteblatt Int. 2012;109:425–30.

19. Newberg AH, Munn CS, Robbins AH. Complications of arthrography. Radiology. 1985;155:605–6.

20. Charalambous CP, Tryfonidis M, Sadiq S, Hirst P, Paul A. Septic arthritis following intra-articular steroid injection of the knee – a survey of current practice regarding antiseptic technique used during intra-articular steroid injection of the knee. Clin Rheumatol. 2003;22:386–90.

21. von Essen R, Savolainen HA. Bacterial infection following intra-articular injection. A brief review. Scand J Rheumatol. 1989;18:7–12.

22. Menkes CJ. Is there a place for chemical and radiation synovectomy in rheumatic diseases? Rheumatol Rehabil. 1979;18:65–77.

23. Taylor WJ, Corkill MM, Rajapaske CAN. A retrospective review of Yttrium- 90 synovectomy in the treatment of knee arthritis. Br J Rheumatol. 1997;36:1100–5.

24. Hedstroem SA, Lidgren L. Septic bone and joint lesions. In: Klippel JH, Dieppe PA, editors. Rheumatology, vol. 4. London: Mosby; 1994. p. 3.1–3.10.

25. Donatto KC. Orthopedic management of septic arthritis. Rheum Dis Clin North Am. 1998;24:275–86.

26. Bueller HR, Agnelli G, Hull RD, Hyers TM, Prins MH, Raskop GE. Antithrombotic therapy for venous thromboembolic disease. Chest. 2004;126:401S–28.

27. Clagett GP, Anderson FA, Geerts W et al. Prevention of venous Thromboembolism. Chest. 1998;114:531S–560S.

28. Fischer M, Ritter B. Prevention of thromboembolism during radiosynoviorthesis. Der Nuklearmediziner. 2006;29:33–6.

29. Gratz S, Goebel D, Becker W. Radiosynovectomy in inflammatory joint disease. Orthopaede. 2000;29:164–70.

30. Gratz S, Goebel D, Behr TM, Herrmann A, Becker W. Correlation between radiation dose, synovial thickness, and efficacy of radiosynovectomy. J Rheumatol. 1999;26:1242–9.

31. Kisielinski K, Bremer D, Knutsen A, et al. Complications following radiosynoviorthesis in osteoarthritis and arthroplasty: osteonecrosis and intra-articular infection. Joint Bone Spine. 2010;77(3):252–7.

32. Mahmoudi M. Therapie der nicht-juvenilen, aseptischen Osteonekrose und des symptomatischen Knochenmarkoedems mit dem Prostazyklinanalogon Iloprost.-Eine MRT-kontrollierte klinische Verlaufsstudie. Düsseldorf. 2009. http://docserv.uni-duesseldorf.de/servlets/.

33. Franchi A, Bullough PG. Secondary avascular necrosis in coxarthrosis: a morphologic study. J Rheumatol. 1992;19:1263–8.
34. Johnson LS, Yanch JC. Calculation of beta dosimetry in radiation synovectomy using Monte Carlo simulation (EGS4). Med Phys. 1993;20:747–754754.
35. Murray K, Dalinka JE, Finkelstein JB. Complications of radiation therapy: adult bone. Semin Roentgenol IX. 1974;1:29–40.
36. Höller U, Hoecht S, Wudel E, Hinkelbein W. Osteonekrose nach Strahlentherapie gynäkologischer Tumoren. Strahlenther Onkol. 2001;177:291–5.
37. Jämsen E, Huhtala H, Puolakka T, Moilanen. Risk factors for infection after knee arthroplasty. J Bone Joint Surg Am. 2009;91:38–47.
38. Jämsen E, Nevalainen P, Kalliovalkama J, Moilanen T. Preoperative hyperglycemia predicts infected total knee replacement. Intern Med. 2010;21:196–201.

Risk of Cancer Induction

10

Cuneyt Turkmen

Contents

10.1 Introduction

Medical use of radiation is now an indispensable part of modern healthcare, and correct risk estimation is essential for justification of radionuclide therapy especially in benign disease. Radiosynoviorthesis is a local intra-articular injection of radiopharmaceuticals for radionuclide therapy. It has now been applied for more than 50 years for treatment of resistant synovitis of the different joints in various inflammatory joint diseases. While there is growing interest in the use of radiosynoviorthesis especially in patients with rheumatoid arthritis and hemophilic synovitis, concerns regarding potential toxicity including a fear of genotoxic effects and carcinogenesis still exist. Throughout this chapter, we will describe specific studies of radiosynoviorthesis and risk of carcinogenesis, touching on strengths and limitations, the need for caution interpretation, and implications for risk assessment.

C. Turkmen, MD
Department of Nuclear Medicine, Istanbul Faculty of Medicine,
Istanbul University, Istanbul 34390, Turkey
e-mail: turkmenc@gmail.com

© Springer International Publishing Switzerland 2015

W.U. Kampen, M. Fischer (eds.), *Local Treatment of Inflammatory Joint Diseases: Benefits and Risks*, DOI 10.1007/978-3-319-16949-1_10

10.2   Radiation Carcinogenesis

Biological effects of ionizing radiation result largely from DNA damage, caused directly by ionizations within the DNA molecule or indirectly from the action of chemical radicals formed as a result of local ionizations. Ordinarily, a high proportion of radiation-induced DNA damage is repaired by the cell, with long-term biological consequences related to a defective DNA repair system [1]. Exposure to ionizing radiation may cause both deterministic and stochastic biologic effects. Deterministic effects are those that typically occur soon after exposure and that increase in magnitude with increasing doses above a threshold dose level. Deterministic doses such as the intended dose on the synovial surface result in cell death. Stochastic effects of radiation typically occur later after exposure, and the probability but not the magnitude of the effects is dose dependent. A threshold dose level for stochastic effects is generally not assumed. Examples of stochastic effects include cancer induction and genetic changes.

Epidemiological studies which attempt to determine the association between radiation exposure and a health outcome have been the main source of information defining the radiation risk. Today, there is also growing interest in biodosimetry techniques to assist in long-term epidemiologic investigations so that radiation-related cancer risks can be estimated as well as possible [2]. These studies have demonstrated that children are considerably more sensitive to the carcinogenic effects of ionizing radiation than adults. Furthermore, children live longer and thus have a larger window of opportunity for expressing radiation damage. Based on epidemiological studies of Japanese atomic bomb survivors and children and infants irradiated for benign diseases such as tinea capitis and skin hemangioma, a distinct pattern of risk for radiation-related tumors has emerged. Dose-related increased risks for cancers of the thyroid gland, breasts, brain, nonmelanoma skin cancer, and leukemia have been observed in adults who were irradiated for benign diseases in childhood [3]. These studies show that the risk of getting cancer rises in a straight line with exposure exceeding doses of 100 mSv. Below that 100-mSv level, however, the risk of cancer induction becomes uncertain.

Both epidemiological and biodosimetric studies of cancer risks associated with exposure to ionizing radiation have some limitations. A major limitation is related to exploring risks to a population from low doses of radiation from high-dose exposure studies, for example, in studies of the survivors of atomic bombing in Japan and in Chernobyl recovery operation workers. There are typically other uncertainties in evaluating the association between radiation exposure and cancer risk. There may be uncertainties in the "transfer" of risk estimated from one population to another, uncertainties in the effect of confounding factors, and uncertainties in the uptake and metabolism of specific radionuclides. Additionally, many factors contribute to the risk for radiation carcinogenesis, some specific to the patient and some of which are specific to radiation treatment. Various kinds of ionizing radiation like electromagnetic (X-rays, gamma rays) or particulate (alpha, beta, neutrons) show remarkable differences of their biological effectiveness. For instance, thyroid cancer has been the single largest health impact of the Chernobyl nuclear disaster, with

6,000 cases identified by 2005, according to an UNSCEAR report, but there is no likelihood of a thyroid cancer being induced by nuclides other than radioiodine [4].

10.3 Risk of Radiosynoviorthesis

Concerns about radiosynoviorthesis include the risks from exposure to ionizing radiation and cancer induction. Since it is a local form of radionuclide therapy, there should be a differentiation of tumor entities and their likelihood of being theoretically induced by radiosynoviorthesis agents. Its safety will depend on the fact which normal structures are in the target of the radiation and the percentage of the dose delivered. Beta-emitting colloidal particles are phagocytized by inflamed hypertrophic synovial tissue, including that part of the synovial lining which lies adjacent to hyaline cartilage at margins. It is therefore an inevitable event that there will be some irradiation of cartilage and subchondral bone during radiosynoviorthesis. Nevertheless, it is established that different tissues (or organs) of the body have different sensitivities for the induction of cancer by radiation. Bone marrow is very sensitive, but hyaline cartilage and muscle tissue tolerate a very high-dose radiation [5]. The dose to the bone marrow in large- or midsize joints is considered negligible owing to the fact that the distance to the radiation source is greater than the mean tissue penetration of radionuclides used for radiosynoviorthesis. Radiocolloid particles which leak out of the treated joints could potentially accumulate in the regional lymph nodes, reticuloendothelial system, bone marrow, and liver [6]. In this context, leakage of beta emitters causes little stochastic exposure especially in the hematopoietic system. No published studies have directly attributed any cancer risk to radiosynoviorthesis. But it is important to recognize how difficult it would be to perform such a study. Because low-dose risks are small and difficult to detect, epidemiological studies with sufficient statistical power would require extremely large populations and careful matching of the subjects in the study to ensure an accurate result.

Epidemiological cohorts continue to play an important role in low-dose radiation research and health risk evaluation in medical exposures as well as other cohorts with high-dose radiation exposure. Unfortunately, there are only two retrospective cohorts published specific to research on cancer incidence among patients treated with radiosynoviorthesis. One small study on the long-term risks of cancer in patients with rheumatoid arthritis who have been treated with Y-90 was reported by Vuorela et al. [7]. It included 143 rheumatoid arthritis patients with a single radiosynoviorthesis of the knee with Y-90, between the years 1970 and 1985, and other rheumatoid arthritis patients not treated with radiosynoviorthesis. The incidence of cancer in patients with and without radiosynoviorthesis was compared with that of the local population during the period starting in 1979 and ending in 1999. Adjusting for age, gender, and calendar period, the study reported no excess cancers in either of the two cohort groups (treated and not treated with radiosynoviorthesis) in comparison with the reference population. More precisely, the standardized incidence ratio for all cancers was 0.6 (95 % confidence interval (CI) 0.3–1.1) for the treated patients and 1.1 (95 % CI 0.9–1.3) for patients not treated with radiosynoviorthesis.

In a larger cohort, Infante-Rivard C et al. studied cancer incidence in patients with rheumatoid arthritis or haemophilic synovitis receiving one or more radiosynoviortheses. Follow-up covered over 25 years and compared the incidence in this group with background rates from the province of Quebec and from other parts of Canada [8]. This study reached similar conclusions with Vuorela et al., but it was substantially larger; it included subjects who had received more than a single treatment and was able to consider quantitative estimates of exposure such as dose and number of radiosynoviorthesis. A total of 4,860 radiosynoviortheses were recorded for the cohort, with subjects receiving between 1 and 16 treatments and a majority (79 %) getting 1 or 2. Treatments were most often administered to the knee joint. Most procedures were done with Y-90 (71 %) or P-32 (29 %). Category-specific rates in this cohort including 2,412 adult patients were compared with rates in similar categories from the general population generating standardized incidence ratios (SIR). No increase in the risk of cancer was observed (SIR 0.96; 95 % CI 0.82–1.12). Additionally, there was no dose–response relationship with the amount of radioisotope administered or number of radiosynoviorthesis.

Epidemiological evidence that low doses of radiation may induce cancer in humans is only available for doses higher than 100 mSv [4]. The effective doses for radiosynoviorthesis given in the dosimetric studies seem to be in the low-dose range (<50 mSv) [9–11]. For example, the effective dose with Re-186 remains approximately 30 times lower than with other treatments such as I-131 in benign thyroid diseases [12]. Also, effective doses in radiological imaging range easily in the same magnitude of 20 mSv, when computed tomography (CT) is used repeatedly. It is almost twice the dose of an abdominal CT image [13]. But that risk is very low overall and may be difficult to measure with epidemiologic techniques.

There have been two cases of acute lymphocytic leukemia reported in hemophilia patients receiving chromic phosphate-32 [14]. Both children, aged 9 and 14 years, had uncomplicated radiosynoviorthesis and developed leukemia within 1 year. Interestingly, both patients had a history of autoimmune disorder, and the interval between exposure and the development of leukemia was less than the expected peak of radiation-induced leukemia. A recent survey of hemophilia treatment centers in the United States (US) identified that approximately 1,100 P-32 radiosynoviortheses were performed in 700 patients with hemophilia, both adults and children, since 1988. While the overall cancer rate in persons with hemophilia is not known, according to one prospective study of malignancy in over 3,000 individuals with hemophilia in the United States, the rate of leukemia was low, less than 1 in 33,000 person-years [15]. Pediatric ALL has a yearly incidence of 1 in 2,500 children under age 15. Estimates from the US national registry would suggest that there should have been 1.5 cases of ALL in the hemophilia population over the last 10 years [16]. It is also kept in mind that there are differences in radiation sensitivity between individuals, depending on their gender, age, genetic factors, lifestyle, and concomitant exposures to other agents. As a consequence of these arguments, the Medical and Scientific Advisory Council of the National Hemophilia Foundation recommends discussion about the risk–benefit ratio of radiosynoviorthesis, including the potential risk of cancer, with all individuals or with their parents considering the procedure, and written informed consent should be obtained which clearly documents that these two cases of malignancy were discussed [17]. Today, Y-90, Re-186, and Er-169 have gained widespread acceptance for radiosynoviorthesis in Europe, and P-32 is no longer mentioned in European guidelines because it has disadvantages such as half-life and high lymphatic transport [18]. Until now, an increased risk of cancer after radiosynoviorthesis with Y-90, Re-186, and Er-169 radiocolloids has not been reported.

Biomarkers that could be used for molecular epidemiological studies in radiation-exposed cohorts are of particular interest. While the validation of potential biomarkers of low-dose ionizing radiation is questioned, there is extensive research in this field [19]. The measurement of chromosome aberrations in peripheral lymphocytes whether stable (balanced translocations) or unstable (dicentrics, ring chromosomes) has been frequently used in studies of patients treated with radiosynoviorthesis. Recently, we studied the cytogenetic analyses such as chromosomal aberration analysis, micronuclei, and sister chromatid exchange as indicators of radiation-induced cytogenetic damage in 38 hemophilic children undergoing radiosynoviorthesis using Y-90 or Re-186 [20, 21]. The results of our studies indicate that high radiation doses, which would induce genotoxic effects, are not obtained by peripheral blood lymphocytes in children after radiosynoviorthesis. Dicentric aberrations are the main interest in these types of studies as the formation of dicentric chromosomes in human peripheral lymphocytes is a specific effect of ionizing radiation [22]. We could not detect any persistent dicentric chromosomal aberrations after the therapy, and there was no statistically significant increase in the number of chromosomal aberrations in children who were treated with Y-90 or Re-186 radiosynoviorthesis. Several studies have confirmed that there was no significant increase in the number of dicentric chromosomes following radiosynoviorthesis in patients who were treated with different radioisotopes [23–25].

Kavakli et al. reported some chromosomal aberrations in 40 patients with hemophilia after radiosynoviorthesis using Y-90 and Re-186. Three months after radioisotope exposure, chromosomal breakages still continued in 21 patients of whom 15 already had chromosomal breakages prior to radiosynoviorthesis, and mean values of chromosomal breakages were not found to be significant. They also pointed out that, after 1 year following the radiosynoviorthesis, four patients had persistent same level chromosomal breakages [26]. Due to the high frequency of chromosomal breakages in the patient group before radiosynoviorthesis and concomitant factors during follow-up, it is difficult to establish a relation between these nonspecific chromosomal breakages and radiosynoviorthesis. Falcon de Vargas et al. carried out a study on 31 hemophilic patients (age range 9–24 years) with no chromosomal aberrations; only nonspecific chromosomal structural changes (breakages) were observed 6 months after Re-186 injection for radiosynoviorthesis, and these changes were reversible after 1 year postinjection [23]. In contrast to these findings, Manil et al. reported a significant cumulative increase in dicentric aberrations 7 days after radiosynoviorthesis in 45 rheumatoid arthritis patients treated with Re-186 [27]. However, as there was no follow-up after 7 days in this study, it is unclear whether this significant increase in dicentrics would be persistent afterward or not.

Even if the relationship of cancer risk with micronuclei is not well substantiated, as is that with chromosomal aberrations, this method has been proven to be useful as a "biologic marker of early effects" in biomonitoring studies on the human population exposed to genotoxic agents. Micronuclei represent small, additional nuclei formed by the exclusion of chromosome fragments or whole chromosomes lagging at mitosis. Micronuclei rates, therefore, indirectly reflect chromosome breakage or impairment of the mitotic apparatus. We have observed mildly increased frequency of micronuclei in the peripheral lymphocytes of hemophilic children 2 days after radiosynoviorthesis in both Y-90 and Re-186 group. But this effect was not persistent in the peripheral lymphocytes of the children in our study and had disappeared at the day 90 control. Kavakli et al. also confirmed these results, and they have reported that there was no significant difference between the hemophilic patients with and without radiosynoviorthesis with respect to micronuclei values [28]. Prosser et al. also analyzed 22 patients with rheumatoid or osteoarthritis of the knee treated with Y-90 silicate, and no significant increase in micronucleus frequency was observed [29].

The long-lasting clinical practice and the lack of any well-documented cases of malignancy resulting from radiosynoviorthesis suggest a very low and acceptable risk compared with the benefit for the patient. The tumor morbidity rate as a result of whole-body irradiation was calculated as 0.4 per 1,000 related to International Commission on Radiological Protection (ICRP) 60 risk data [30], and the genetic radiation risk related to United Nations Scientific Committee on the Effects of Atomic Radiation (UNSCEAR) data was described as being several orders of magnitude below 1 per 1,000 [31]. On the other hand, because of the complexity of biomonitoring of genotoxicity, we need further investigations to understand the radiation effects in untargeted living systems exactly. Furthermore, radiation effects are thought to be cumulative, which is of particular importance in children diagnosed with hemophilia. Debate continues on what cumulative level is acceptable for cancer risks for the patients need recurrent radiosynoviorthesis due to chronic disease. Patients should understand that radionuclide therapies should only be performed when the effectiveness to be gained justifies the potential harm. Decision-making about radiosynoviorthesis should include a thorough conversation between patients and their doctors regarding the benefits and risks of the procedure. While the benefits of radiosynoviorthesis outweigh the risks of developing subsequent cancers, the presence of such risks could implicate the need for further investigation into methods of minimizing the radiation dose delivered to joint and surrounding tissues.

References

1. Little JB. Radiation carcinogenesis. Carcinogenesis. 2000;21(3):397–404.
2. Simon SL, Bouville A, Kleinerman R. Current use and future needs of biodosimetry in studies of long-term health risk following radiation exposure. Health Phys. 2010;98(2):109–17.
3. Kleinerman R. Cancer risks following diagnostic and therapeutic radiation exposure in children. Pediatr Radiol. 2006;36 Suppl 14:121–5.

4. UNSCEAR. Sources, effects and risks of ionizing radiation. New York: United Nations Scientific Committee on the Effects of Atomic Radiation, United Nations; 2006. Available at: www.unscear.org/unscear/en/publications/2006_1.html. Accessed Aug 2014.

5. Martin LM, Marples B, Lynch TH, et al. Exposure to low dose ionising radiation: molecular and clinical consequences. Cancer Lett. 2013;338(2):209–18.

6. Turkmen C. Safety of radiosynovectomy in hemophilic synovitis: it is time to re-evaluate! JCD. 2009;01:29–36.

7. Vuorela J, Sokka T, Pukkala E, et al. Does yttrium radio-synovectomy increase the risk of cancer in patients with rheumatoid arthritis? Ann Rheum Dis. 2003;62(3):251–3.

8. Infante-Rivard C, Rivard GE, Derome F, et al. A retrospective cohort study of cancer incidence among patients treated with radiosynoviorthesis. Haemophilia. 2012;18(5):805–9.

9. Klett R, Puille M, Matter HP, et al. Activity leakage and radiation exposure in radiation synovectomy of the knee: influence of different therapeutic modalities. Z Rheumatol. 1999;58:207–12.

10. van der Zant FM, Jahangier ZN, Moolenburgh JD, et al. Radiation synovectomy of the ankle with 75 MBq colloidal 186 rhenium sulfide: effect, leakage, and radiation considerations. J Rheumatol. 2004;31:896–901.

11. Grmek M, Milcinski M, Fettich J, Brecelj J. Radiation exposure of hemophiliacs after radiosynoviorthesis with 186Re colloid. Cancer Biother Radiopharm. 2007;22(3):417–22.

12. International Commission on Radiological Protection (ICRP). Radiation dose to patients from radiopharmaceuticals. Publication 53. Ann ICRP. 1987;18:1–4.

13. Brenner DJ, Hall EJ. Computed tomography: an increasing source of radiation exposure. N Engl J Med. 2007;29(357):2277–84.

14. Dunn AL, Manco-Johnson M, Busch MT, Balark KL, Abshire TC. Leukemia and P32 radionuclide synovectomy for hemophilic arthropathy. J Thromb Haemost. 2005;3:1541–2.

15. Ragni MV, Belle SH, Jaffe RA, Duerstein SL, Bass DC, McMillan CW, Lovrien EW, Aledort LM, et al. Acquired immunodeficiency syndrome-associated non-Hodgkin's lymphoma and other malignancies in patients with hemophilia. Blood. 1993;81:1889–97.

16. Dores GM, Devesa SS, Curtis RE, et al. Acute leukemia incidence and patient survival among children and adults in the United States, 2001–2007. Blood. 2012;119(1):34–43.

17. MASAC Recommendations Regarding Radionuclide Synovectomy. MASAC recommendation number 194, National Hemophilia Foundation. 2010. Available via DIALOG: http://www. hemophilia.org/Researchers-Healthcare-Providers/Medical-and-Scientific-Advisory-Council-MASAC/All-MASACRecommendations/Recommendations-Regarding-Radionuclide-Synovectomy. Accessed Aug 2014.

18. Clunie G, Fisher M. EANM procedure guidelines for radiosynovectomy. Eur J Nucl Med. 2003;30:BP12–6.

19. Léonard A, Rueff J, Gerber GB, Léonard ED. Usefulness and limits of biological dosimetry based on cytogenetic methods. Radiat Prot Dosim. 2005;115(1–4):448–54.

20. Turkmen C, Ozturk S, Unal SN, et al. The genotoxic effects in lymphocyte cultures of children treated with radiosynovectomy by using yttrium-90 citrate colloid. Cancer Biother Radiopharm. 2007;22(3):393–9.

21. Turkmen C, Ozturk S, Unal SN, et al. Monitoring the genotoxic effects of radiosynovectomy with Re-186 in paediatric age group undergoing therapy for haemophilic synovitis. Haemophilia. 2007;13(1):57–64.

22. Rodrigues AS, Oliveira NG, Gil OM, Leonard A, Rueff J. Use of cytogenetic indicators in radiobiology. Radiat Prot Dosim. 2005;115:455–60.

23. Falcon de Vargas A, Fernandez-Palazzi F. Cytogenetic studies in patients with hemophilic hemarthrosis treated by 198Au, 186Rh, and 90Y radioactive synoviorthesis. J Pediatr Orthop B. 2000;9(1):52–4.

24. Voth M, Klett R, Lengsfeld P, et al. Biological dosimetry after yttrium-90 citrate colloid radiosynoviorthesis. Nuklearmedizin. 2006;45(5):223–8.

25. Fernandez-Palazzi F, Caviglia H. On the safety of synoviorthesis in haemophilia. Haemophilia. 2001;7 Suppl 2:50–3.

26. Kavakli K, Cogulu O, Aydogdu S, et al. Long-term evaluation of chromosomal breakages after radioisotope synovectomy for treatment of target joints in patients with haemophilia. Haemophilia. 2010;16:474–8.
27. Manil L, Voisin P, Aubert B, et al. Physical and biological dosimetry in patients undergoing radiosynoviorthesis with erbium-169 and rhenium-186. Nucl Med Commun. 2001;22:405–16.
28. Kavakli K, Cogulu O, Karaca E, et al. Micronucleus evaluation for determining the chromosomal breakages after radionuclide synovectomy in patients with hemophilia. Ann Nucl Med. 2012;26(1):41–6.
29. Prosser JS, Izard BE, Brown JK, et al. Induction of micronuclei in peripheral blood lymphocytes of patients treated for rheumatoid or osteoarthritis of the knee with dysprosium-165 hydroxide macroaggregates or yttrium- 90 silicate. Cytobios. 1993;73(292):7–15.
30. International Commission on Radiation Protection. ICRP-60: recommendations of the ICRP. Ann ICRP. 1991;21:1–3.
31. Brenner W. Radionuclide joint therapy. In: Eary JF, Brenner W, editors. Nuclear medicine therapy. New York: Informa Healthcare; 2007. p. 21–44.

Baker's Cysts: A Relevant Contraindication?

11

Rigobert Klett

Contents

11.1 Anatomy, Etiology, and Pathogenesis

Popliteal cysts, also called Baker's cysts, are fluid-filled masses in the popliteal fossa. Based on anatomical aspects, three types of popliteal cysts can be distinguished: synovial, meniscal, and ganglion cysts [1]. Relative to radiosynoviorthesis (RSO) in particular, the synovial popliteal cysts are of interest. In the group of synovial popliteal cysts, the most frequent one has its origin in a bursa located at the medial head of the gastrocnemius muscle. Together with another bursa located beneath the tendon of the semimembranosus muscle, a communicating gastrocnemio-semimembranosus bursa can be found. Contemporarily this communicating bursa is the most frequent origin of a popliteal cyst [2]. At the level of the medial femoral condyle, the posterior capsule of the knee shows weaker regions with the possibility of herniations of the articular synovial membrane. In this area the gastrocnemio-semimembranosus bursa usually communicates to the knee [3]. Cysts communicating to the knee joint also are called secondary cysts, instead of primary cysts without any communication to the knee joint. Most of the primary cysts are found in

R. Klett
ÜBAG für Nuklearmedizin, Hanau – Frankfurt – Offenbach – Gießen,
Standort Gießen, Paul-Zipp-Straße 171-173, 35398 Gießen, Germany
e-mail: rigobert.klett@radiol.med.uni-giessen.de

© Springer International Publishing Switzerland 2015
W.U. Kampen, M. Fischer (eds.), *Local Treatment of Inflammatory Joint Diseases: Benefits and Risks*, DOI 10.1007/978-3-319-16949-1_11

children and develop before the age of 15. In adults almost all popliteal cysts are secondary cysts associated to different knee joint pathologies. For example, meniscal tears are responsible for the development of these cysts in 71–82 % [4], degenerative cartilage lesions in 30–60 %, and anterior cruciate ligament insufficiency in 30 % [5, 6]. The prevalence rate of popliteal cysts in knee magnetic resonance imaging was between 5 and 19 % [5, 6]; using ultrasound as imaging modality, Mödder reported a prevalence rate of 25 % in 980 RSO of the knee joint [7].

11.2 Hydrostatic Aspects, Valvular Mechanism

Pressures in the knee joint and a corresponding Baker's cyst were measured by Jayson and Dixon [8] in 12 patients with rheumatoid arthritis. Simultaneously arthrograms of the knee joint were performed. In all cases the contrast media passed from the knee into the cyst. In the extended position of the knee and the heel elevated on a small block, the intracystic pressures (mean 72.2 mmHg) were significantly higher than the intra-articular pressures (mean 13.6 mmHg). Cyst squeezing resulted in an increased pressure in the cysts up to several hundred mmHg but showed no significant pressure increase in the knee joint. Measurement under knee flexion (45° and 90°) was performed in five knees with the result of decreasing cyst pressure in all cases. Two cysts could be reduced into the knee with flexion and manipulation. In one cyst a valvular mechanism could be demonstrated. After squeezing the distended knee, the knee pressure decreased below its initial value, and the cyst pressure increased in comparison to the initial pressure. Similar results are found by Lindgren [9]. Based on those results, Jayson and Dixon [8] discussed two possible forms of valve mechanisms. One model resembles a ball valve due to large quantities of fibrin within the cyst blocking the connection to the knee under high pressure (Fig. 11.1). Alternatively, a Bunsen-type valve is possible, consisting of a narrow curved passage in which walls collapse under direct cyst pressure.

In an anatomical study, Rauschning [3] found a communication between the knee joint and Baker's cysts in 58 of 108 knees. The communication becomes progressively wider with increasing flexion as the gastrocnemius tendon was pulled away from the femoral condyle. On extension the capsule of the knee joint was compressed between the tendon and the femoral condyle. This result can explain the decreasing pressure in the Baker's cysts under knee flexion. Because of the anatomical structure of the communication between the cyst and knee, Rauschning contradicted the hypothesis of a valve mechanism of the Bunsen type. Considering the observation of Pindler [10] who could empty all 14 popliteal cysts into the joint cavity during anterior synovectomy in spite of containing fibrin masses, Rauschning also contradicted the hypothesis of a true valve mechanism of the ball type. Instead, he interpreted the closing mechanism as a functional action concerning both directions and excluded a unidirectional valve mechanism.

Some other study results are also in contradiction to a unidirectional valve mechanism. Wilson et al. [11] found that air, injected in a popliteal cyst, promptly passed into the joint even if it is not possible to empty the cyst into the joint. Maudsley and Arden [12] described an activity trespassing into the knee joint after injection of

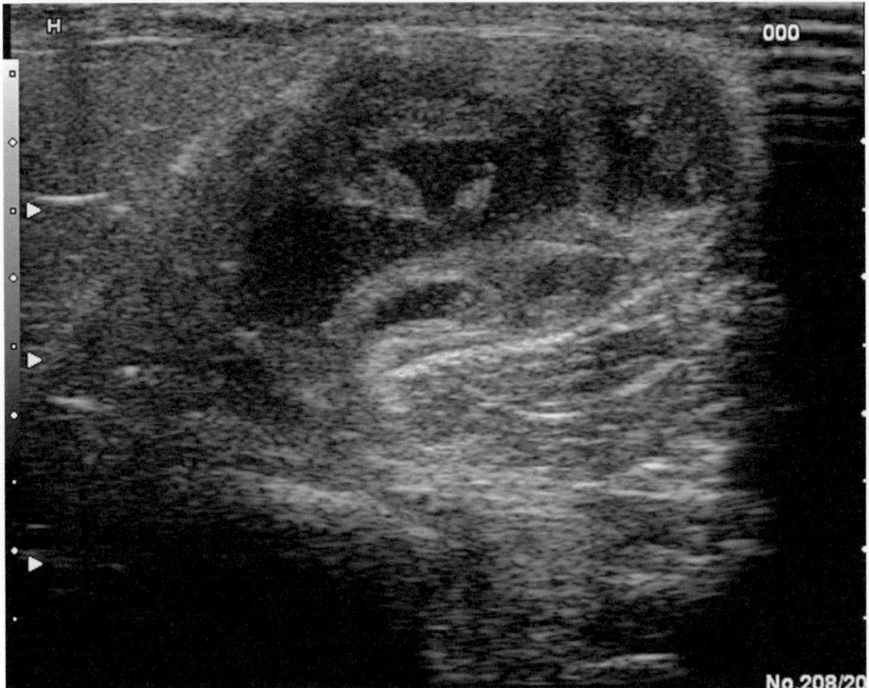

Fig. 11.1 Example of a Baker's cyst with a possible ball valve mechanism due to large quantities of fibrin within the cyst as assumed by Jayson and Dixon [8]

yttrium into a popliteal cyst. In ten patients Smith et al. [13] measured activity distribution into Baker's cysts after RSO of the knee using single-photon emission computed tomography (SPECT) and found 0–40 % of the activity in the cysts. Up to 46 h, repeated measurements over time showed no activity accumulation; during this time the patients were confined to bed.

11.3 Treatment Results of Baker's Cysts After RSO

Up to now, only a small number of studies described the effect of RSO of the knee joint to Baker's cysts. Grahame et al. [14] treated 15 patients: 13 showed a Baker's cyst, and in 2 cases the cyst extended into the calf. In 4 of the 13 patients, the cyst disappeared. The time difference of control and treatment was between 6 and 11 months.

Topp et al. [15] described a study of 112 RSO of knee joints; the treatment results were controlled up to 5 years. Twelve patients had a popliteal cyst or synovial rupture or both, and in all cases the lesion disappeared or decreased in size.

In a prospective study of 150 RSO of knee joints with Baker's cyst, Mödder [16] reported on 87 disappeared cysts after the first RSO. Another 57 cysts disappeared after a second RSO. Time difference of control and treatment was not mentioned.

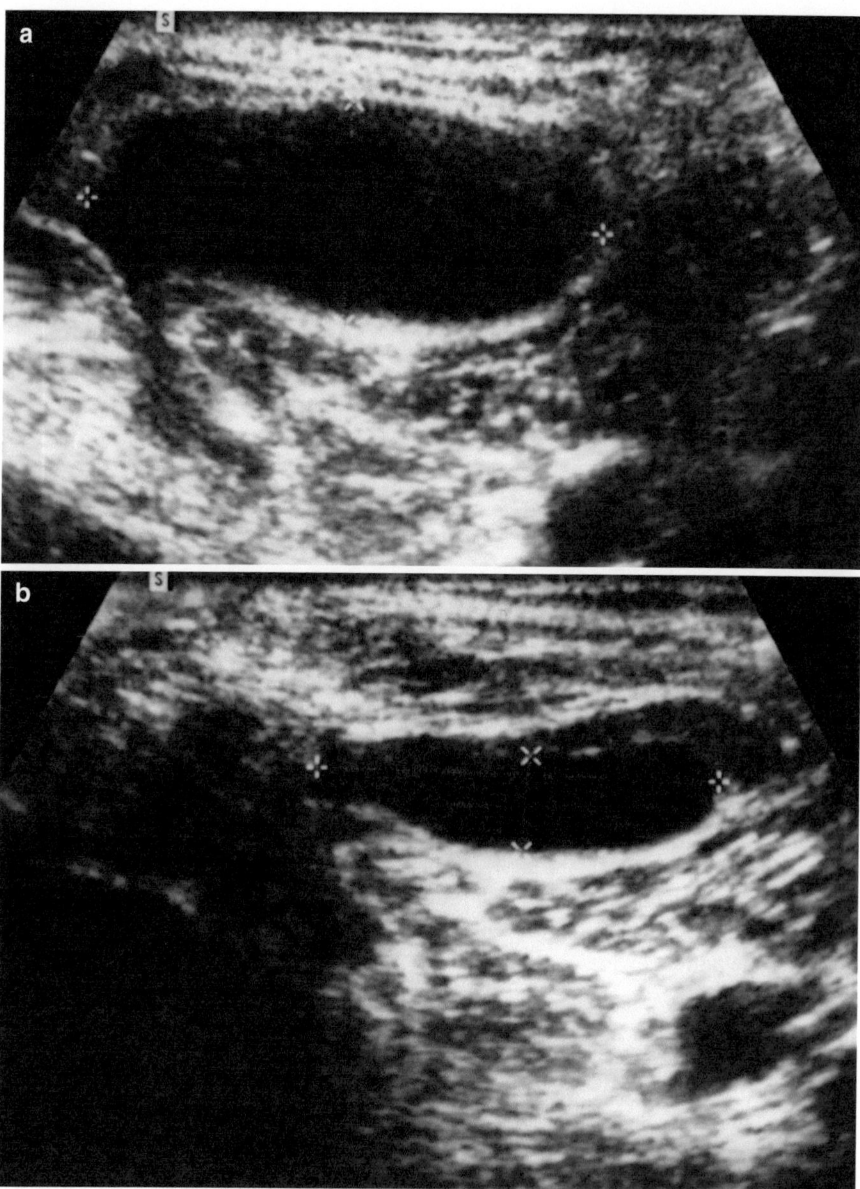

Fig. 11.2 Volume reduction of a Baker's cyst due to RSO of the knee joint. (**a**) Baker's cyst before RSO. (**b**) Baker's cyst 5 months after RSO

Our own data of 60 RSO with Baker's cysts in 45 patients showed a significant reduction of the median cyst volume of 73 % after a median follow-up of 6 months (Fig. 11.2). In 25 % of cases the cyst disappeared, and in 55 % the volume was reduced, whereas in 20 % the volume increased [17].

Table 11.1 Activities in knee joint fluid and Baker's cyst fluid, respectively, 12 days after RSO and decay-corrected activities 48 h after RSO

	Aspirated activity/ml [kBq]	Decay-corrected aspirated activity/ml 48 h after RSO [kBq]	Activity/100 ml 48 h after RSO [kBq]	Injected activity 48 h after RSO [kBq]
Patient 1 (joint puncture)	3	40	4,000	137,000
Patient 2 (cyst puncture)	<1	<13	<1,300	120,000

11.4   Risk Estimation for Baker's Cyst Rupture

Neither of the above-cited treatment studies reported any complication corresponding to Baker's cyst. Nevertheless, Asavatanabodee et al. [18] described a Baker's cyst rupture in 5 of 133 treated knee joints; time difference between RSO and rupture was not mentioned. In addition, Davis and Jayson [19] reported two cases of a knee joint rupture occurring 43 and 63 days after RSO.

The most severe complication would be the rupture of a Baker's cyst directly after RSO, draining the activity into the calf. Therefore, for risk estimation not only the probability of cyst rupture but also the quantity of activity present within the fluid inside the cyst needs to be assessed. Standard of care mandates the immobilization of the knee joint for 48 h after RSO, so cyst rupture based on external stress can be expected earliest after the end of this immobilization period.

Because of aggravation of symptoms and recurrence of effusion, a puncture of the knee joint in one patient and of the Baker's cyst in another patient had to be performed in our institution to exclude infection 12 days after RSO with the possibility of activity measurement in the aspirated fluid. Table 11.1 depicts the results of activity per ml aspirated fluid, decay-corrected activity per ml 48 h after RSO of the aspired fluid, and activity in the whole lumen of the knee joint and Baker's cyst due to the injected activity 48 h after RSO. In addition, for risk estimation, the activity per 100 ml fluid 48 h after RSO as a worst case was calculated due to the activity in the aspirated fluid.

The results show a huge difference between the calculated activity inside the joint due to the injected activity and the measured activity of the aspirated fluid with decay correction. This difference can be explained by the fast phagocytosis of the injected radiocolloids into the synovial membrane. Therefore, also in the unlikely case of a rupture of the Baker's cyst, the emptied activity into the calf is very low, and a distinctive damage of the popliteal and calf tissue should not be expected.

11.5   Discussion

Initially Baker's cyst was classified as an absolute contraindication for RSO of the knee joint because of some reports of spontaneous rupture, especially corresponding to patients with recurrent joint effusion [20–22]. Even today some authors still classify Baker's cyst as an absolute contraindication [23]. Nevertheless, 20 years ago, Mödder [16] introduced a more differentiated view of the topic. He suggested the use of ultrasound to differentiate between Baker's cyst with and without a valve mechanism and classified only Baker's cysts with valve mechanisms as an absolute contraindication.

Considering the results described in Sect. 11.2, a unidirectional valve mechanism is very unlikely and can be classified as irrelevant relating to the risk of cyst rupture directly after RSO. In general, activity will be injected into the knee in the extended position. Under this condition, the study of Rauschning [3] in combination with the results of Smith et al. [13] suggested either an immediate homogenous activity distribution into the cyst or a lack of activity distribution, depending on the special anatomical situation of the patient. In particular an activity and fluid trapping within Baker's cyst resulting in increasing pressure are very unlikely under the condition of joint immobilization. Nevertheless, Asavatanabodee et al. [18] described a rupture of Baker's cyst after RSO in five cases. Because knee joints were not immobilized in their study, this reported complication is not transferable to today's situation. The additionally reported knee joint rupture by Davis and Jayson [19] cannot be pointed out as a direct consequence of the RSO because of the long time interval between RSO and rupture (43 and 63 days, respectively).

The risk of damage to the soft tissue due to released activity is established as low, based on the low free fluid activity estimated 48 h after RSO (see Sect. 11.4). The few reports of knee joint RSO in the presence of a synovial or cyst rupture without any damage of the soft tissue [15, 18] support this risk assessment.

In addition, in an inquiry of 260 nuclear medicine physicians and 20 medical liability insurances about the kind and frequency of complications corresponding to RSO between 1998 and 2003, no rupture of a Baker's cyst was reported [24].

Overall, a Baker's cyst should not be classified as a relevant contraindication for RSO of the knee joint. Rather with respect to the reported positive effect of RSO in knee joints with Baker's cyst [14–17], RSO should be included into a multimodal therapy regime of Baker's cyst.

Consistent with the above considerations, current literature and especially guidelines classify only a ruptured Baker's cyst as a contraindication [25–27]. Even

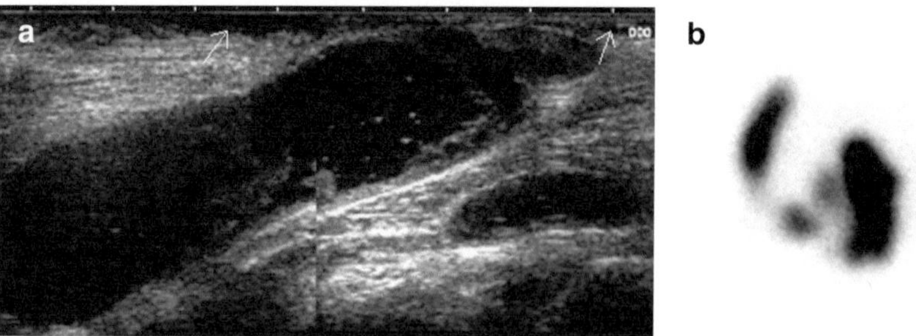

Fig. 11.3 (a) Ultrasound with possible fluid leakage from the Baker's cyst into the surrounding tissue (*arrows*). (b) Joint cavity scintigraphy excludes leakage from the Baker's cyst

though risk can be assumed as low, a ruptured Baker's cyst should be classified as a relevant contraindication based on the very limited and only theoretical data. Therefore, it is recommended to exclude a rupture of an existing Baker's cyst before RSO by ultrasound. In case of doubt a joint cavity scintigraphy with Tc99-labeled colloids should be performed to exclude leakage from the cyst into the surrounding tissue (Fig. 11.3a, b).

Literature

1. Malghem J, Vandenberg BC, Lebon C, et al. Ganglion cysts of the knee: articular communication revealed by delayed radiography and CT after arthrography. Am J Roentgenol. 1998;170:1579–83.
2. Fritschy D, Fasel J, Imert J-C, et al. The popliteal cyst. Knee Surg Sports Traumatol Arthrose. 2006;14:623–8.
3. Rauschning W. Anatomy and function of the communication between knee joint and popliteal bursae. Ann Rheum Dis. 1980;39:354–8.
4. Stone KR, Stoller D, De Carli A, et al. The frequency of Baker's cysts associated with meniscal tears. Am J Sports Med. 1996;24:670–1.
5. Miller TT, Staron RB, Koenigsberg T, et al. MR imaging of Baker cysts: association with internal derangement, effusion and degenerative arthropathy. Radiology. 1996;201:247–50.
6. Sansone V, De Ponti A. Arthroscopic treatment of popliteal cyst and associated intra-articular knee disorders in adults. Arthroscopy. 1999;15:368–72.
7. Mödder G. Radiosynoviorthese, [^{224}Ra] Radiumtherapie und Röntgenstrahlentherapie. In: Zeidler H, Zacher J, Hiepe F, editors. Interdisziplinäre klinische Rheumatologie. Berlin: Springer; 2001. p. 361–77.
8. Jayson MIV, Dixon AJ. Valvular mechanisms in juxta-articular cysts. Ann Rheum Dis. 1970;29:415–20.
9. Lindgren PG. Gastrocnemio-semimembranosus bursa and its relation to the knee joint. III: pressure measurements in joint and bursa. Acta Radiol Diagn Stockh. 1978;19:377–88.
10. Pindler IM. Treatment of the popliteal cyst in the rheumatoid knee. J Bone Joint Surg. 1973;55B:119–25.
11. Wilson PD, Eyre-Brook AL, Francis JD. A clinical and anatomical study of the semimembranosus bursa in relation to popliteal cyst. J Bone Joint Surg. 1938;20:963–84.
12. Maudsley RH, Arden GP. Rheumatoid cysts of the calf and their relation to Baker's cysts of the knee. J Bone Joint Surg. 1961;43B:87–9.
13. Smith T, Shawe DJ, Crawley JCW, et al. Use of single photon emission computed tomography (SPECT) to study the distribution of 90Y in patients with Baker's cysts and persistent synovitis of the knee. Ann Rheum Dis. 1988;47:553–8.
14. Grahame R, Ramsey NW, Scott JT. Radioactive colloidal gold in chronic knee effusions with Baker's cyst formation. Ann Rheum Dis. 1970;29:159–163.
15. Topp JR, Cross EG, Fam AG. Treatment of persistent knee effusions with intra-articular radioactive gold. Can Med Assoc J. 1975;112:1085–9.
16. Mödder G. Die Radiosynoviorthese. Nuklearmedizinische Gelenktherapie (und –diagnostik) in Rheumatologie und Orthopädie. Warlich, Meckenheim; 1995
17. Klett R, Stahl B, Steiner D, et al. Radiosynoviorthese des Kniegelenkes zur nicht invasiven Therapie von Baker-Zysten. Nuklearmedizin. 2003;42:A128.
18. Asavatanabodee P, Sholter D, Davis P. Yttrium-90 radiochemical synovectomy in chronic knee synovitis: a one year retrospective review of 133 treatment interventions. J Rheumatol. 1997;24:639–42.
19. Davis P, Jayson MIV. Acute knee joint rupture after yttrium 90 injection. Ann Rheum Dis. 1975;34:62–3.

20. Bandilla K. Radionuklidbehandlung von Gelenkerkrankungen. Nuklearmediziner. 1979;4:292–9.
21. Makoski H-B, Strötges MW, Rau R, et al. Radionuklidtherapie rheumatischer Gelenkerkrankungen. Therapiewoche. 1982;32:4805–12.
22. Stock C, Puhl W, Georgi P. Radiosynoviorthese. Orthopadische Praxis. 1983;8:583–4.
23. Rehart S, Arnold I, Fürst M. Die konservative Lokaltherapie des entzündeten Gelenks. Lokal-invasive Therapieformen. Z Rheumatol. 2007;66:382–7.
24. Kampen WU, Matis E, Czech N, et al. Serious complications after radiosynoviorthesis. Survey on frequency and treatment modalities. Nuklearmedizin. 2006;45:262–8.
25. Kampen WU, Voth M, Pinkert J, et al. Therapeutic status of radiosynoviorthesis of the knee with yttrium [90Y] colloid in rheumatoid arthritis and related indications. Rheumatology. 2007;46:16–24.
26. Brenner W. Radionuclide joint therapy. In: Eary JF, Brenner W, editors. Nuclear medicine therapy. New York: Informa Healthcare; 2007. p. 21–44.
27. Clunie G, Fischer M, EANM. EANM procedure guidelines for radiosynovectomy. Eur J Nucl Med. 2003;30:BP12–6.

Summary

Willm Uwe Kampen and Manfred Fischer

Reasons for inflammatory joint disease are as variable as possible strategies to treat its clinical signs like joint effusion, pain and restricted joint motion. These symptoms lead to a significant decrease of the patient's quality of life and should be satisfactorily treated.

In patients with systemic rheumatoid diseases, with severe osteoarthritis or even with acute joint effusion after trauma or surgery, the inflammation of the synovial membrane, i.e. synovitis, is the reason for the above-mentioned inflammatory complaints. Thus, synovitis is the main target of any treatment modality which might be chosen from the large armamentarium available today.

This book gives a review over both systemic pharmacotherapies and local treatment options, the latter consisting of conservative, surgical and nuclear medical therapies. Since there is a large spectrum of clinical appearances in different patients, a "golden standard" of treatment cannot exist. Thus, different medical specialists like rheumatologists, orthopedists, surgeons, nuclear medicine physicians and others should develop the tailored treatment for the individual patient from an interdisciplinary approach.

Especially due to this interdisciplinarity, everyone who is engaged with the treatment of inflammatory joint diseases should be aware of both the basic effects and possible side effects of the different therapies. This should influence the decision how to treat the individual patient.

We hope that this book will help to decide about the proper treatment approach and to weight the desired therapeutic effects against possible risks to choose the best therapy with an optimal outcome.

W.U. Kampen
Nuklearmedizin Spitalerhof, 8, Hamburg 20095, Germany
e-mail: kampen@nuklearmedizin-spitalerhof.de

M. Fischer (✉)
Institute of Radiology, Radiation Therapy and Nuclear Medicine, Friedrich-Ebert-St., D-34117, 55 Kassel, Germany
e-mail: finukskk@aol.com

© Springer International Publishing Switzerland 2015

W.U. Kampen, M. Fischer (eds.), *Local Treatment of Inflammatory Joint Diseases: Benefits and Risks*, DOI 10.1007/978-3-319-16949-1

Moreover, we hope that the chapters dealing especially with radiosynoviorthesis might be helpful in recurring discussions on possible risks and side effects of this classical nuclear medicine therapy. Based on a substantial knowledge, the reader should be able to set the true indication for this treatment or even to refuse it in patients where there is no perspective for any clinical benefit or when possible risks prevail the expected effects.